Teaching Hospitals and the Urban Poor

Teaching Hospitals and the Urban Poor

Eli Ginzberg

with the assistance of
Howard Berliner
Miriam Ostow
Panos Minogiannis
and J. Warren Salmon

The Eisenhower Center for the
Conservation of Human Resources
Columbia University

Yale University Press
New Haven and London

Printed in the United States of America

Library of Congress Cataloging-in-Publication Data
Ginzberg, Eli, 1911–
Teaching hospitals and the urban poor / Eli Ginzberg ; with the assistance of Howard Berliner et al.
p. cm.
Includes index.
ISBN: 0-300-08232-0 (cloth : alk. paper)
1. Academic medical centers—United States. 2. Urban poor—Medical care—United States. 3. Medical care—United States—Finance. 4. Hospitals, Teaching—United States. 5. Poverty—United States. 6. Urban Health Services—United States.
RA981.A2 G493   2000
362.1′1′0973 21
(DNLM)100941728   00-028294

A catalogue record for this book is available from the British Library.

The paper in this book meets the guidelines for permanence and durability of the Committee on Production Guidelines for Book Longevity of the Council on Library Resources.

10   9   8   7   6   5   4   3   2   1

To Giselle
Good friend and companion in my later years
With affection and appreciation

Contents

Preface

Once again my coworkers at the Eisenhower Center, Columbia University, and I are deeply indebted to the Pew Charitable Trusts, which underwrote the present study following our completion of their earlier-sponsored study on *Tomorrow's Hospital: A Look to the Twenty-first Century* (Yale University Press, 1996).

A word about our title. One or more of the experts (see below) who reviewed our draft manuscript questioned the inclusion of "urban poor." After careful deliberation we decided not to drop this phrase on the ground that the less-than-intimate relationship between the academic health centers and the urban poor was one of our critical findings.

Having noted the help that we received from our expert readers, we are listing them below (and the positions they held as of that time) and acknowledging our deep appreciation of their many corrections and additions as well as the participation of most of them at Columbia during a day-long meeting that helped us to sharpen and refine our analysis: Professor Lawrence Brown, Head, Policy and Management Division, Columbia University School of Public Health; Dr. Spencer Foreman, President and CEO, Montefiore Medical Center, Bronx, New York; Dr. Robert Lawrence, Associate Dean, School of Hygiene and Public Health, Johns Hopkins University; Dr. Mitchell Rabkin, President, CareGroup, Boston; Dr. Rosemary Stevens, Stanley I. Sheerr Endowed Term Professor in Arts and Sciences, Department of History and Sociology of Science, University of Pennsylvania; Mr. James Tallon, Jr., President, United Hospital Fund, NYC; Dr. Bruce Vladeck, Department of Health Policy, Mt. Sinai Hospital, NYC.

A word about chapter 4, "Challenging the AHCs to Change." The initial focus of this book was planned to center on "The Health of the Public (HOP)" program which Pew, Rockefeller, and R. W. Johnson Foundations supported from 1986 to 1996. While we were discussing our new research plan with the Pew staff we were alerted by them that the current foundation sponsors, Pew and R. W. Johnson, were likely to terminate their HOP program support shortly, which, in fact, they did. This helps to explain both our focus in chapter 4 on HOP as well as our selective treatment of the demonstration.

Two additional long-term members of the Eisenhower Center staff must be singled out for their major assistance: Charles Frederick undertook the stylistic review of the draft manuscript and made our analyses easier for the reader to follow. And Shoshana Vasheetz, our long-term stalwart secretarial right hand, once again stayed on top of my multiple handwritten drafts that she alone was able to decipher.

Teaching Hospitals and the Urban Poor

Introduction

As the title of this book suggests, our study takes up questions concerning academic health centers (AHCs) in urban settings. We attend especially to the circumstances of the twenty-five or so leading research-oriented AHCs. This cohort of AHCs (see table) is largely concentrated along the East and West Coasts, from Boston to Durham, North Carolina, and from San Diego to Seattle, but also includes representation from the Midwest and the South. We need to take particular notice of the derailment of the Clinton health reform proposal in September 1994 because it is a crucial condition for this study. A consequence of this failure is that lower-income groups, the poor, and the uninsured will continue to face difficulties as they wait for broadened access to the health care system.

The leading research-oriented AHCs enter the present moment with many strengths. They are staffed with large faculties of outstanding clinicians and researchers. They are in close relationship with one or more owned (or affiliated) hospital centers, frequently of 750 to 1,000 beds, and they have annual budgets sometimes in excess of $1 billion. Yet at the same time, the AHCs have clearly

The Top 25 Research-Oriented AHCs in the United States
(1997 grants by the National Institutes of Health)

East

Johns Hopkins University School of Medicine, Baltimore (1)

University of Pennsylvania School of Medicine, Philadelphia (3)

Yale University School of Medicine, New Haven (4)

Columbia University College of Physicians and Surgeons, New York (11)

University of Pittsburgh School of Medicine, Pittsburgh (13)

University of North Carolina School of Medicine, Chapel Hill (14)

Harvard Medical School, Boston (18)

Albert Einstein College of Medicine, Yeshiva University, New York (22)

New York University School of Medicine, New York (25)

West

University of California–San Francisco School of Medicine, San Francisco (2)

University of Washington School of Medicine, Seattle (6)

Stanford University School of Medicine, Stanford (7)

University of California–San Diego School of Medicine, La Jolla (12)

University of California–Los Angeles School of Medicine, Los Angeles (16)

University of Colorado Health Science Center School of Medicine, Denver (20)

Midwest

Washington University School of Medicine, St. Louis (5)

University of Michigan Medical School, Ann Arbor (9)

Case Western Reserve University School of Medicine, Cleveland (10)

University of Chicago Pritzker School of Medicine, Chicago (19)

University of Minnesota–Minneapolis Medical School, Minneapolis (24)

South

Duke University School of Medicine, Durham (8)

University of Alabama School of Medicine, Birmingham (15)

Baylor College of Medicine, Houston (17)

University of Texas Southwest Medical Center–Dallas (21)

Vanderbilt University School of Medicine, Nashville (23)

Note: Ranking by total dollar value of grants

Source: National Institutes of Health Annual Report 1997, Award Data Section, Washington, D.C.

entered stormy waters. Admissions for inpatient care at the AHCs dropped precipitously in the early 1980s and have never recovered, in part because of the growth of community hospital capabilities and changing patterns of medical treatment allowing for ambulatory care. Other factors include advances in surgical techniques and in anesthesia allowing same day, in-and-out surgery. Compounding this downward trend in hospital revenues has been a radical decline in patients' average length of stay, thereby accelerating the buildup of unused hospital beds in most metropolitan areas and intensifying fiscal pressures on many AHCs. The AHCs, meanwhile, have been increasingly confronted by aggressive purchasers seeking large discounts.

Additional challenges have surfaced for AHCs located in regions where managed care plans made the most rapid progress in enrolling the below-65 population. San Diego, Los Angeles, and the Twin Cities are the best examples of this situation; Boston is a more recent one. The managed care plans were not content to reduce the number of members referred to hospitals for inpatient care and to limit the stays of those who were hospitalized; they also looked for less-costly alternatives to the AHCs altogether when authorizing enrollees to obtain inpatient care.

The leading research-oriented AHCs had long priced their services at 25–30 percent above the charges of community hospitals. This higher rate was necessary to ensure that they could cover the high costs of their more seriously ill patients as well as the extra unfunded costs associated with their special missions. These unfunded costs included supporting young investigators not sufficiently advanced to procure their own research money, sponsoring intramural clinical investigations, covering the difference between medical students' tuition expenses and their total education costs, and providing an alternative source of funding for charity patients.

Charity patients account for about 1 in 7 admissions to public AHCs and 1 in 20 to nonprofit AHCs.

What is the simple definition of this institution we are discussing, the academic health center? According to common usage, an AHC consists of a medical school and one or more health professional schools, such as dentistry, nursing, or public health. These schools are joined to one or more affiliated teaching hospitals that are under common ownership or closely aligned with the medical school. About 60 percent of all AHCs are sponsored by the state in which they are located, and the rest operate predominantly under nonprofit auspices.

Although the leading medical schools on the East Coast — Harvard, Yale, Columbia, the University of Pennsylvania, and Johns Hopkins — originate in the eighteenth and nineteenth centuries, this book is generally concerned with issues and circumstances arising since the early to mid-1960s. It was at the beginning of this period that the federal government initiated large-scale funding grants to enable the nation's existing medical schools to increase enrollments and to encourage states and private universities to establish new medical schools.

Congress passed Medicare and Medicaid in 1965. This legislation made large amounts of federal and state funding available for expanded medical and hospital care for the elderly and for many of the nonelderly poor. In the same year Congress amended the long-standing immigration and naturalization statutes, permitting thousands of graduates of foreign medical schools to obtain their residency training in the United States. Most of these graduates remained to practice medicine and today account for about 1 in 4 of all practicing physicians in this country.

What makes for the logic in the title of this work — *Teaching*

Hospitals and the Urban Poor? We first should explain whom we mean when we say "the urban poor." Are they people with an income below the federal level of poverty or slightly above, approximately 125 percent of the poverty level? Are they the uninsured? What about the poor who are eligible for Medicaid? The urban poor in the context of this book include all of these groups. This is admittedly a broad category, but one with a commanding, common characteristic. These people encounter at least small—but most often great—difficulty in obtaining regular access to the range, quality, and continuity of health care services available to most Americans.

Certainly many of the urban poor have needed improved access to both routine and more specialized medical care. But most AHCs have not been particularly responsive. AHCs in general have not considered the provision of primary care services to be an integral part of their mission. Accordingly they have sought to limit the amount of charity care that they provide to large numbers of the urban poor who lack proper health insurance coverage. In fact, AHCs have been overwhelmingly driven by internally generated values and goals. The AHC agenda has been concisely and successfully aimed at advancing medical knowledge and techniques that will lead to more effective treatment of patients, reduced morbidity, and increased years of healthy life.

Yet, as will be explained, the AHCs were significantly linked with the urban poor even in the pre-Medicare–Medicaid era, during which time the centers admitted a certain number from this population to carry out their educational mission. Perhaps the two are linked even more strongly now, however, in this era of Medicaid managed care when the AHCs face diminished inpatient lists and must reassess their patient relationships. This population might be a means toward mitigating the future decline in inpatient revenues. Further, as the AHCs confront growing pressures to expand ambulatory clinic facilities for training medical students and residents, the urban poor again become an important element in answering a current need. Although location has been and remains a critical determinant of where people seek care, we must remain aware of the considerable variability in the proximity of concentrations of the urban poor to AHCs even within the same metropolitan area. The principal teaching hospitals of many of the oldest—and often most distinguished—of the AHCs, especially along the eastern seaboard, were created in the heart of their respective cities close to where the poor were heavily concentrated and to whose needs they catered. This variation is even greater among diverse metropolitan centers.

Because this volume focuses on the AHCs and the urban poor during the past three decades, we need to take particular note of the major role that Medicare and Medicaid played in transforming the financial well-being of all AHCs. The new funds made available from this legislation converted many charity and part-paying patients into full-paying patients. This legislation also made special funding available to the AHCs for graduate medical education and provided funding for the professional care that some clinical staff members gave to patients who were not admitted by a private physician. Medicare and Medicaid also disbursed liberal funding for the future capital outlays of teaching hospitals.

This volume follows on the heels of an earlier study by the Eisenhower Center, published as *Tomorrow's Hospital: A Look to the Twenty-first Century* (Yale University Press, 1996). Not only is this other study of chronological importance, it is also germane to the subject of the present book. The Pew Charitable Trusts (which sponsored this book), in association with the Rockefeller Foundation and later with the Robert Wood Johnson Foundation, made grants in the years 1986–1996 to competing AHCs for the purpose of stimulating them to initiate curriculum reforms. These reforms were to be aimed at establishing or broadening existing AHC offerings in population-based medicine. The grants were also intended to encourage the AHCs to enter into partnerships with their low-income neighbors to improve the urban poor's access to more and better ambulatory care services, both preventive and therapeutic.

The Eisenhower Center staff was finalizing discussions with the Pew Charitable Trusts staff to undertake a study of these community partnerships sponsored by the foundations' Health of the Public program when the Pew staff suggested that we also direct our attention to Medicaid managed care. Their thinking was that the new and rapidly growing program was likely to alter drastically the provision of medical care to the poor in the years ahead.

The analysis in this book is centered primarily on the changing relations between the AHCs and the urban poor subsequent to the transforming events of the 1960s, particularly the passage of Medicare and Medicaid. For this analysis to be fully informed, however, we believed it necessary to provide a brief account of the complex changes in the structure and functioning of the U.S. health care financing and delivery system as a result of the World War II — hence chapter 1 on "The Impact of World War II on U.S. Medicine."

Chief among the transformations beginning in this period has been the growing role of the federal government—witness such initiatives as the large-scale funding for biomedical research via the National Institutes of Health. Another intervention of long-lasting consequence was the decision of the War Labor Board in

1942 and subsequent action by the Treasury Department to establish a special tax subsidy for both the providers and the recipients of group health insurance benefits. As of 1997 these actions, although helping to expand enormously the number of people with private health insurance coverage, have been estimated to result in an annual subsidy of $100 billion. Witness, too, the passage of the Hill–Burton Act (1946), which made federal funds available for the first time to assist small- and medium-sized communities to build or upgrade community hospitals. And we should not forget that as an ancillary consequence of World War II military service, many Americans gained a greatly enhanced appreciation for the potential of modern medical care. Unequivocally stated, World War II, coinciding with the arrival of penicillin launched the U.S. medical care system on a new trajectory.

Chapter 2, "How Medicare Changed the AHCs," examines how Medicare transformed the financial circumstances of the nation's leading research-oriented AHCs. Once financially constrained institutions, they now found themselves relatively awash in money because of this largess. Medicare's liberally funded graduate medical education was one new source of funds, and its cost-plus-reimbursement policy was another. Additionally, the AHCs found relief from earlier pressures to admit charity patients to meet their teaching obligations since, with the passage of Medicare, most patients became patients available for teaching purposes. Moreover, a substantial increase in federal funds for residency training started with Medicare. All of these new money streams for education were directed only to the AHCs' major teaching hospitals, whereas the cost-plus-payment policy applied to all hospitals.

The medical school component of the AHC benefited as well, beginning in 1963 with the introduction of the 13-year cycle of federal funding for medical schools. Adding to the improved budget picture for medical schools was their modification in staffing strategy, beginning largely in the 1980s. Under this scheme, the leading AHCs appointed a vast number of new clinical professors under terms that required them to earn their salaries and benefits and to contribute 10 to 15 percent to the institution's coffers. Chapter 3, "Changes in the Physician Supply," looks first at consequences resulting from the 1963 initiatives to provide direct federal funding for expanding the medical school output, and then to Medicare reimbursement starting in 1966, helping the AHCs and other teaching hospitals to cover the costs of training and employment of residents. Also discussed in this chapter is the phenomenon of the tens of thousands of international medical graduates attracted to the United States for residency training, enabling them later to practice in this country. A few facts begin to illustrate the qualitative and quantitative changes in the physician supply. First, federal funding was provided to enlarge the enrollments of existing medical schools and to stimulate the establishment of new medical schools. As a consequence, the annual output of U.S. medical graduates doubled from about 8,000 to 16,000 between the early 1960s and the early 1980s. Second, Medicare provided liberal funding for residency training, including its proportional share of the cost of stipends to residents, determined essentially from the ratio of Medicare patients to all patients admitted. Most residents decided to pursue subspecialty training, which became the predominant choice, particularly among those who were trained at the nation's leading research-oriented AHCs. Last, the number of international medical graduates admitted to the United States and permitted to remain here to practice numbered approximately 175,000 in 1998.

Chapter 3 also considers efforts by the federal and state governments to counteract the emphasis on subspecialty training by encouraging the training of more generalists. This chapter takes a broad look at the ways in which Congress, the medical leadership, and the public at large have approached the complex issue of the desirable size of the physician supply through the years.

As mentioned, our original plan had been to undertake an in-depth study of the experience of the AHCs that had been awarded Pew-Rockefeller-Johnson grants to assess the centers' experience with so-called community partnerships with the urban poor. Chapter 4 has a considerably broadened policy perspective, however, reflecting the greater compass to which our research brought us. With their funding intervention, the sponsoring foundations had wished to influence a shift in the curriculum of medical schools more in the direction of population medicine and away from the schools' prior—almost exclusive—preoccupation with patho-physiology. This chapter focuses on the factors that both facilitated and impeded this change of direction. We seek to identify in particular how the flow of funds into the AHCs created multiple power centers in the affluent clinical departments that individually and collectively had more dollars under their control than the funds under the direct jurisdiction of the dean. We opened the scope of our analysis to review and assess the manifold objectives of the foundations' public health initiatives as they developed. These goals over time went considerably beyond curricular reform and community partnerships to involve public policy issues and financing. We also consider such unanticipated consequences as the establishment of an informal network of mostly younger investigators. These investigators were linked by a common concern with restructuring the efforts of the AHCs away from their almost exclusive focus on the delivery of high-tech medicine and toward including the improvement of the health status of their low-income neighbors. We further recognized the need to identify, at least briefly, other changes in the health care marketplace. Some of these evolutions are likely to have significant longer-term consequences for the future welfare of both the AHCs and the urban poor because of the need of many if not most AHCs to capture more referrals from among the Medicaid population. What might be the impact of the rapid growth of Medicaid managed care for the health care services available to enrollees? The AHCs need to reevaluate how they can expand their access to ambulatory care sites. One way to realize this goal is to provide more care for their low-income neighbors.

Chapter 5, "The Impacts of Managed Care," selectively reviews the major reasons for the rise and growth of managed care plans, particularly after 1980. We investigate the growing enrollments of Medicaid-eligible individuals into this new system of financing and providing health care to the urban poor. We use 1980 as the starting point because the preceding 15 years had been uniquely characterized by an almost total unlinking of dollar controls from the expanding use of medical services. The two principal payers— employers and government—almost without review or questioning paid all bills submitted by providers of care to patients with private or public health insurance coverage. Hence it is not at all surprising that managed care or some similar control mechanism would arise to reestablish dollar controls over medical services delivered to insured patients. What is surprising is that the period of disconnection had been tolerated for a decade and a half and continued for yet another decade in many parts of the country.

The first half of this chapter explores the rise of the independent physicians association/network model that emerged in southern California. Shifting fee-for-service insured enrollees into a managed care plan achieved overall savings of approximately 15 percent. Fueling their growth was the stock market boom and the willingness of the capital markets to make large advances to the rapidly expanding, for-profit managed care plans. Next we take up the vulnerability of the AHCs in rapidly expanding managed care environments. With charges that are 30 percent higher than those at comparable facilities, the AHCs were at a competitive disadvantage given the managed care plans' determined efforts to restrict admissions of their enrollees for inpatient hospital care, especially to high-cost institutions.

The second half of the chapter focuses on the more recent explosive growth of Medicaid managed care and the efforts to enroll considerable numbers of low-income persons not previously eligible for public coverage. We take up the question of the larger industrialized states, including California, Illinois, and New York, all of which continue to encounter major hurdles in their attempts to transfer the urban poor rapidly into Medicaid managed care. We conclude by exploring reasons that allowed many of the nation's leading AHCs to distance themselves from the urban poor after the enactment of Medicare and Medicaid. This discussion is juxtaposed with a description of the market forces that are now leading at least some of the same AHCs to explore how they can establish new relationships with the urban poor whose care, especially hospital care, can fill some of their vacant beds and contribute to their bottom line.

Our concluding chapter, "The Next Decade," emphasizes how well-positioned financially the leading research-oriented AHCs were in the first two decades after the enactment of Medicare and

Medicaid. Bolstered by broad public support for their high-tech plans, AHCs were able to redefine and aggressively pursue their these goals through their increasingly expensive programs of education, research, and patient care. At the same time, however, these AHCs further distanced themselves from the urban poor. The availability of large numbers of international medical graduates provided a substantial health care workforce for many low-income, particularly immigrant, neighborhoods. And presently, although the rapid growth of managed care enrollments has sent a warning shot across the bows of even the most prestigious AHCs, most of them, through a series of innovations and cost-containment efforts, have thus far been able to stay on course. Also to be brought into the equation is President Bill Clinton's promise of an order of magnitude rise in federal support for their future research budgets and the prospects of the fulfillment of this promise. In addition, we assess important trends and events connected with the explosive growth of managed care and the greater challenges that AHCs may face as a result of this revolution. The Congressional Budget Office predicts a continuing steep rise in national health expenditures, expected to exceed $2 trillion annually by 2007. The combined government outlays for health care in 1998, which include the large tax subsidy for private health insurance coverage, approximately $100 billion, exceed $600 billion.

Finally we explore briefly what might be possible if the number of the uninsured and the underinsured continues to grow: the American people may at long last seek to tackle two long unmet challenges. The first is to provide a system of essential health care coverage for all citizens and permanent residents. The second might be to moderate the steep increases in government expenditures for health care by forcing the more affluent to use their own dollars if they want more choices of providers and more-expensive procedures. We also briefly address important policy challenges that affect the AHCs specifically and that grow out of the pressing need to reduce excess hospital capacity. We look at questions relating to the future supply of physicians while also considering possible actions to increase the number of underrepresented minorities, primarily African American and Hispanic medical school graduates.

In the end we return to the challenge posed in the title of this book. With the implementation of Medicare and Medicaid, the leading AHCs could set their sights almost exclusively on pushing back the frontiers of high-tech medicine, while at the same time many were becoming estranged from the urban poor. Will the changes in the health care marketplace now under way in the financing and delivery of medical care bring about a closer realignment between the AHCs and the poor?

1
The Impact of World War II on U.S. Medicine

Although this chapter focuses on the important changes in the structure and function of U.S. medicine between World War II and the passage of Medicare and Medicaid, we begin by identifying key interactions between the leading urban academic health centers and their low-income neighbors. We will use 1910 as a starting date, when the young educator Abraham Flexner completed the first major report on U.S. medical education under the sponsorship of the Carnegie Foundation for the Advancement of Teaching and with the support of the AMA. Flexner's recommendations were twofold. First, he recognized the urgent need for the United States to reduce significantly the number of medical schools from around 160 to 39 to enhance the quality of medical education. Second, but not secondarily, he believed that the nation's medical school faculties should be strengthened and enlarged so that both the courses they taught and the medical diagnoses and treatments they provided would be firmly undergirded by a scientific foundation based on modern biology.

We should recall that some of today's leading AHCs began their operations in the nineteenth century and a few even as early as the eighteenth. Established largely with philanthropic funding, these AHCs were products of major teaching hospitals that combined with medical schools with a primary goal of providing hospital care and comfort to the neighborhood sick and injured, particularly to the victims of the periodic epidemics that afflicted so many urban residents. Not until the late nineteenth and early twentieth centuries did increasing numbers of the middle- and upper-income population begin to use the acute care hospital.

By the mid-1920s Flexner's reforms were largely in place, and a number of the nation's leading medical schools had allied themselves with a well-functioning acute care hospital to form an academic health center. These early AHCs had a small full-time faculty, relying on volunteer physicians to provide most of the clinical instruction. Their research activity was limited, and funding was often provided by an affluent physician on the staff or one of his wealthy patients. The AHC students were predominantly undergraduates. Most of these students, after earning their M.D. and completing a one-year internship and passing the licensing examination, would enter practice.

Many neighborhood practitioners were willing to provide hours of uncompensated care in the clinics and on the wards of teaching hospitals. This was particularly the case at AHCs that operated under public auspices and provided charity care as part of their mission and responsibilities. Until the advent of penicillin, which occurred at about the same time as the start of World War II, not even the AHCs could do much for many severely ill and injured patients other than to provide comfort care. Their limited capabilities largely explain why many of the nation's leading teaching hospitals were able to meet their budgets by charging patients, often 40 to 50 in a single ward, only $5 per day. When patients themselves could not make payments, the charges were covered by philanthropic funds and by the extra costs assessed against private patients. An important difference between then and now was the dependence of the medical school on its affiliated hospital to admit reasonable numbers of charity patients. Students in training—medical students, interns, and the relatively small numbers of graduates who sought advanced (specialized) training—needed access to these patients, because paying patients were not then generally available to them.

The United States experienced striking advances in the health of its people during the first decades of the twentieth century, but these gains had relatively little to do with the improved diagnoses and therapies of curative medicine. Instead they mostly reflected such public health advances as the elimination of many infectious and contagious diseases; improvements in the water supply; better sanitation; the improved handling of food products, including milk pasteurization; a better understanding of nutrition; and a host of other highly successful interventions. Another way of describing the relatively limited scale and scope of the nation's health care sector when the United States entered World War II is to recall that the total expenditure for the nation's health care sector was approximately 4 percent of the nation's quite modest gross domestic project (GDP). At the end of the 1930s the GDP was no larger than it had been at the beginning of the decade because of the depth of the depression and the slow recovery that followed.

Flexner's report set U.S. medicine on its scientific path for the next three decades. During this time the quality of medical education had also been greatly improved, as many inadequate schools were closed, and the surviving schools raised their requirements for admission and graduation. Accompanying these reforms were selected advances in radiology, pathology, surgery, and other specialties, and in pharmaceuticals. But the substantial gains in the health of the American people during these decades mostly reflected gains in the public health arena. Progress in public health was itself closely related to advances in the educational level of Americans and their rising standard of living, at least before the onset of the Great Depression. It is thus ironic that medical schools did not teach their students more about public health issues. But overall the United States made tremendous progress in curative medicine in the half-century following the war and ultimately emerged as the world's leader in high-tech medicine.

After the nation went to war, many army enlistees revealed that they had had no previous contact with physicians, hospitals, or clinics. Their first encounter with a modern health care system occurred after they were in uniform, and most responded favorably about the care that they received. Approximately 15 million enlistees and draftees saw service during the war in the army (which included the air corps) or the navy (which included the marines), and all had access to the military health care system. Additionally, several million dependents of the uniformed forces also had some exposure to the medical departments of the army and navy. Together, people in the armed services and their dependents made up about 1 in 6 Americans.

The experiences of the millions who were in the uniformed services during the war, and especially the several hundred thousand battle casualties who were returned to the United States for medical or surgical treatment, produced a widespread, generally positive perception of the contribution that an effectively functioning health and hospital system could make to the well-being of both the armed forces and Americans in general. Wounded World War II soldiers who received immediate medical treatment on the battlefield from a medical corpsman had a 93 percent chance of recovery when finally discharged from a U.S. army hospital.

The active participation of the United States in World War II also brought changes to the health care system at home. The army and navy called on about 40 percent of active physicians who had been engaged in providing health care services to the civilian population. To compensate, at least in part, for the reduced availability of physicians, most remaining practitioners stopped making house calls and saw patients in their office or at a hospital clinic. The federal government also intervened and enrolled medical students in the reserves, paying them a stipend and encouraging medical schools to accelerate their teaching programs to enable graduates to join the armed services more quickly.

Of long-term significance to the U.S. health care system was the importance that the army attached to its commissioned medical officers who entered the service as board-qualified specialists. The army made a commitment to provide the highest possible level of medical care to its troops, especially those seriously injured in battle. As part of this obligation the army organized its general hospitals by specialty center. Facing shortages of specialists among its commissioned physician ranks, the army offered higher rank, more pay, and better assignments to those who were board certified. As the war began to wind down, Congress passed the GI Bill with its multiple monetary and educational benefits for those who had earned an honorable discharge. Impressed by the military's emphasis on specialty certification, many medical officers took advantage of this opportunity to enter or complete their residency training. Underscoring this attention to specialty care was the army policy of matching the type of care that the wounded or otherwise disabled returnee required with the general hospital best able to provide it. The only other criterion that played a role in the assignment process was locating a specialized hospital closest to the patient's home.

The growth in the number of Americans with health insurance was another outcome of U.S. involvement in the war. Although the beginnings of private health insurance under the Blue Cross movement is usually set as 1929 in Dallas, Texas, the total number of Americans with health insurance rose to no more than 15 percent of the population by the outbreak of World War II. Only after the United States entered the war do we see a considerable increase in the number of insured persons. The trade unions petitioned the War Labor Board in 1942 for permission to negotiate for health care benefits in collective bargaining with employers despite the board's earlier ruling against wage increases. The unions persuaded the board that acquiring health care benefits would not be inflationary. In addition, the Treasury Department decided that employers and employees could "pay for such health benefits using pretax income. This subsidy accelerated the number of beneficiaries in employer health care benefit programs. As of November 1997, health care economist and Princeton University professor Uwe Reinhardt estimated that the current annual value of the tax subsidy approximated $100 billion. This subsidy partially explains continued U.S. corporate involvement with health insurance despite growing conflicts with disgruntled current and retired employees. A second explanation is the general reluctance of private business to expand the role of the government in this area. Third, the tax subsidy is especially valuable to those in higher earning brackets.

U.S. involvement in World War II had two additional repercussions on the nation's health care sector. The first concerned federal support for biomedical research. The federal government had taken the lead during the war to finance important research and development projects, with the atom bomb being the most important example. With prompting from Chicago activist Mrs. Albert Lasker and other proponents of expanded federal funding for research into heart disease, stroke, and cancer, the government entered into a policy of active support for biomedical research after the war. By 1998 this support approximated $14 billion. Bolstering the AHCs in their efforts to secure these funds is the $20 billion that they receive annually in corporate investments to speed the development of new and improved health care techniques and products. AHCs with intellectually strong faculties and ongoing access to philanthropic funds are well positioned to compete successfully in the peer-reviewed process to obtain support from the enlarged National Institutes of Health program for biomedical research.

The passage of the Hill-Burton Act in 1946 was the war's other important consequence affecting health care financing and delivery. This legislation made significant federal funds available for the first time to small and medium-sized communities to build or upgrade their community hospital. In the absence of such assistance these areas might otherwise not have been able to attract or retain physicians who would be willing to practice locally. The depression and the war had resulted in a serious backlog in hospital construction, making the new financing of Hill-Burton all the more important. Senate Republican leader Robert Taft played a key role in the passage of this legislation. We should not underestimate the importance of this initiative to expand the access of Americans to hospital care. Hill-Burton was a departure for the federal government; Congress had never before become directly involved in financing hospital care services for the American people. Although this assistance was restricted to smaller and medium-sized communities, it is an important development nevertheless.

At the same time, the lack of activity in other areas likewise has affected the restructuring of the U.S. health care system. The failure of Congress to increase the supply of physicians is one such example. In the decade after the war various states and nonprofit sponsors established new medical schools. In 1948 Social Security administrator Oscar Ewing recommended that President Truman seek federal funding for expanding the physician supply. However, in the face of strong opposition from the AMA to direct federal funding for medical schools, Congress failed to act.

Universal health care coverage is another example. Shortly after the war, Truman, with the support of liberal Democrats in Congress, sought to put universal health insurance on the congressional docket. This effort did not succeed, largely because of strong opposition from the AMA. Also, most trade unions that had won private health insurance benefits from their employers saw little gain from a new system of tax-based insurance coverage. Moreover, a growing number of employers were comfortable with the health care benefits that they had recently introduced and saw no point in involving the federal government. Waiting in the wings were the private insurance companies that had belatedly begun to recognize the new profit opportunities once they learned how to sell health care coverage to private employers. Not to be overshadowed were Blue Cross and Blue Shield, both of which had a major stake in the continuation of the status quo.

One way to assess the long-term impacts of World War II on

the development of the U.S. health and hospital system is to point to the lack of changes in overall structure and functioning. Most physicians continued to practice as generalists, primarily as solo entrepreneurs or as members of small groups. The steady growth of hospital insurance, followed by health insurance coverage for physicians' fees, removed the two barriers that had reduced or blocked access to hospital care for many of the uninsured and the poor. The steady rise in the earnings of nurses and other health personnel and supporting staff in the two decades following the end of World War II also boosted the cost of hospital care. Among other consequences, these increases presented a much greater challenge to philanthropists to continue to provide free and below-cost care to many patients. Also, hospital trustees felt more pressure to find the additional capital funds that their staffs required to keep the hospital at the forefront of diagnostic and treatment capabilities.

But much of the post–World War II health care system was upbeat. Most physicians ready to return to or enter private practice encountered expanded opportunities. College graduates with an interest in attending medical school found reduced admission barriers, primarily because of the much-lowered birth rate of the 1930s. One of the more interesting developments was the continuing leadership role of the AMA and its state affiliates, despite the growth of specialist societies that were attracting more members as advances in medical knowledge and techniques created opportunities for more physicians to limit their practice to a single specialty.

With hindsight we could conclude that World War II had passed without changing the U.S. health care system except for diagnostic and treatment advances that significantly extended the potential contributions of curative medicine to the well-being of the sick and injured who had access to the mainline system. But as we clarify in following chapters, critical unsolved issues pressed for attention and action. Particularly important was to ensure continued access to physician and hospital care for the retired population, which no longer enjoyed employer-financed hospital care coverage. Another issue was the number of physicians that the nation needed to train and how these additional training costs would be covered. A third crucial problem was the trade-off between redirecting U.S. medical practice toward the specialties while many patients continued to need generalist care.

2
How Medicare Changed the AHCs

In passing the Balanced Budget Act of 1997 Congress decided to "save" $115 billion from 1998 to 2002 primarily by reducing payments to the providers of services to elderly and disabled Medicare beneficiaries. This will not be the last time that Congress will have to struggle with introducing radical changes in the Medicare structure, as other factors are demanding attention. The government has already restructured the Medicare Trust Fund. The baby-boom generation becomes eligible for Medicare beginning in 2011. The House of Representatives turned down a Senate amendment to raise the age of eligibility for Medicare from 65 to 67. We are hearing repeated warnings from federal experts that future Medicare expenditures are heading upward at a rate that requires radical action.

These difficulties notwithstanding, Medicare unquestionably represents an outstanding success story. Through this program some 38 million elderly and disabled people have broader and deeper access to health care. Medicare also brought about much expanded financing of the nation's AHCs, which, in turn, helped the research community to push back the frontiers of biomedical knowledge. In addition, Medicare and related legislation provided the funding for the training and employment of a vast number of medical and surgical specialists, enabling the United States to move to the forefront in the delivery of acute care medicine.

To take up the many questions involving reform proposals for Medicare as the nation moves into the twenty-first century, we need to look at the overall impact of Medicare to date. How did this legislation, enacted in 1965, in concert with later modest amendments to the program, reshape the U.S. medical care system? We must also consider some of the critical questions that must be resolved if Medicare is to continue to contribute to the health and well-being of the elderly in the early decades of the twenty-first century.

The challenge is great even for those of us who lived through those feverish years that preceded the passage of Medicare to reconstruct the intensity with which the leadership of the AMA fought the pending legislation. The nation had increasingly become aware of the major shortcoming of private health insurance that the United States had come to rely upon in the post–World War II decades. These arrangements had provided good health and hospital coverage for most employed workers and their dependents, but they left large numbers of the retired elderly at serious risk when they were most in need of hospital coverage. True, Congress had at the end of the 1950s sought to respond to this challenge by providing federal funding to the states to enable their welfare commissioners to help pay the bills of the impecunious elderly admitted for expensive hospital care. But the Kerr-Mills legislation and earlier approaches had not worked very well; most of the needy elderly had no prior experience with the welfare system, so they continued to shun it—even tough they lacked hospital coverage.

The leadership of the AMA decided in 1963 to withdraw its long-term opposition to direct federal support for medical education. It chose instead to concentrate its lobbying efforts to defeat the pending Medicare effort that was making steady progress in Congress, headway that accelerated once Lyndon Johnson scored his overwhelming victory in the 1964 presidential election. The leadership of the AMA decided to leave no stone unturned to derail Medicare as a tax-supported system of health insurance coverage for the elderly. AMA leaders believed that, if passed, this legislation would rapidly advance the U.S. health care financing and delivery system toward socialism.

The all-out efforts of the AMA to derail Medicare failed. What's more, Congress at the same time passed a parallel bill, Medicaid. This legislation provided substantial federal financial support—between 50 and 80 percent—to supplement state spending on the health care needs of citizens and permanent residents whose incomes fell below the federal poverty level. Representative Wilbur Mills of Arkansas, the head of the House Ways and Means Committee, and colleagues from other low-income states organized widespread support for this bill.

Related to this discussion was the issue of universal health care coverage, whose advocates expected that the passage of both Medicare and Medicaid would also help remove the final hurdles blocking their goal. They believed that federal health care coverage for women and children would likewise be approved soon and that the nation would be that much closer to essential health coverage for all, an achievement they believed to be possible during the following decade.

Once Medicare had been signed into law early in 1965, President Johnson went out of his way to reassure the leaders of the AMA that its passage definitely would not disturb the long-term relations between patients and their physicians. He emphasized that the only difference would be in the form of the federal government picking up all future bills. To reassure the leadership of the AMA and the American Hospital Association that the federal government would adopt an inobtrusive stance, Medicare payments would be executed by regional Blue Cross plans and other health care organizations that were currently the key intermediaries in processing the bills generated by private health insurance coverage. Federal agencies would not be directly involved.

Years later it is easy to recognize that the passage of Medicare, along with subsequent developments affecting the scope and administration of the statute, had revolutionary consequences for the future functioning and operations of the health care sector. These went far beyond accomplishing Medicare's major objective of providing enhanced access for the elderly to mainline medical and hospital care under conditions in which most of their acute care costs would be covered by the federal government. The passage of Medicare had long-term consequences for the accelerated growth of total U.S. health expenditures. In the three decades following the passage of this legislation, these expenditures exploded from $41 billion to $1 trillion annually. Even after correcting for inflation, this expansion still represents about a fourfold increase in real dollars per capita. Medicare's inflationary nature was evident from the start, because it was essentially an unrestricted fee-for-service program to doctors and a cost-plus reimbursement program to hospitals.

When Medicare began, the hospital sector accounted for about one-third of total annual U.S. health care outlays, the single largest component among the major expenditure categories. With private health insurance accounting for only about 70 percent of their annual revenues, most hospitals—both large teaching institutions as well as smaller community hospitals—operated under difficult financial circumstances. They were often short of funds to upgrade their facilities and equipment, not to mention augmenting their professional and support staffs.

Most hospitals operated either at or near the break-even point. They had to pay close attention not to admit more than a small number of patients who would be unable to pay their bills. Operating so close to the margin, many teaching hospitals were hard pressed to increase the size of their residency and fellowship programs. Further, they could compensate those in training only with modest stipends, and this arrangement placed residents under pressure to earn additional money in their limited free time. Many of the leading AHCs had to address yet another financial challenge that they could not meet while operating on the fiscal edge: large numbers of their most gifted staff members wanted to shift from part-time to full-time so that they could better focus their energies and improve their productivity (as well as enhance their status and prestige by becoming professors).

The passage of Medicare and subsequent reimbursement policies largely helped to transform the financial circumstances of the nation's leading AHCs, particularly those at the forefront of teaching large numbers of residents and fellows and pursuing a wide array of research projects, basic and applied. Medicare's reimbursement policies went a long way toward improving the financial position of most AHCs. Not only did these policies create a reimbursement system based on the participating hospital's operating costs, they also included payment of approximately an additional 10 percent to help cover the hospital's capital costs. The revenue demands on the large teaching AHCs were further eased after the passage of Medicare because they no longer had to admit considerable numbers of charity patients to meet their teaching responsibilities. In fact, many of the formerly poor elderly, who were earlier treated for free only because of teaching needs, were now covered by Medicare and still remained available for teaching purposes. Moreover, not long after the implementation of Medicare the traditional large wards, where scores of poor patients had been hospitalized in a single wing, gave way by federal mandate to semiprivate accommodations. The teaching hospitals could then raise their room costs accordingly, generating a considerably larger flow of revenue, most of which came from the federal and state governments and private health insurance plans.

One of the most important of the new financing arrangements under Medicare was the payment that the federal government made to hospitals for the direct and indirect costs connected with the operation of residency and fellowship training programs. Shortly after the passage of Medicare, the stipends for residents were increased to an amount approaching a living wage. The new reimbursement arrangements also made payments to the teaching hospital for staff supervision of the rapidly expanding number of residents. As this figure increased, sometimes even by an order of magnitude, much of the routine supervision of the bedridden became the responsibility of the junior and senior residents. This new staff organization made it considerably easier for many attending physicians to accept and treat larger numbers of private patients. Moreover, residents came to play an expanded role in the teaching and supervision of medical students during their junior and senior clinical years. Medical school deans have estimated that residents currently provide more than 60 percent of the clinical supervision of junior and senior medical students.

The sizable state as well as federal funding being made available to voluntary and public hospitals under Medicare and Medicaid took much pressure off the leading urban voluntary teaching hospitals to continue to admit uninsured or underinsured patients. With reasonably clear consciences, the staffs of some AHCs and other leading teaching hospitals referred such patients to public institutions whose primary mission was to care for the uninsured and the poor. The urban poor continued to seek care at an AHC emergency room or clinic, because many states required all hospitals to operate an emergency room on a round-the-clock, daily basis, to care for all who sought treatment and to admit those who were seriously ill.

Various phenomena attest to the impact of Medicare reimbursement policies on the nation's leading hospitals. When the long-term rise in patient admissions reversed and began to decline by the early 1980s, the proportion of hospital costs to total health care costs had increased from approximately 30 to more than 40 percent, and on a much larger patient base. But another important shift also warrants attention. When Medicare was first implemented, about two-thirds of all the revenues of the nation's 80-plus medical schools consisted primarily of federal and state government funding. The professional staffs contributed through practice plan earnings only a small amount toward their medical school budget, approximately $56 million annually or slightly more than 6 percent of a total revenue of $880 million. Thirty years later, with a sizable increase in the number of AHCs from about 80 to more than 120, the totals and the proportionate contributions looked very different. In 1997 hospital and practice plan income accounted for just over half of an almost $35 billion revenue.

From these figures we first should notice the explosive growth in the total revenues of the nation's medical schools since the mid-1960s, from about $900 million to $35 billion. Even after correcting for inflation this reflects a dramatic, nearly tenfold increase. More detailed inspection of the financial reports of medical schools reveals a striking decline in the proportion of government funding in the past three decades. By the mid-1990s this funding had fallen to the low 30 percent range, less than half of what it was in the mid-1960s. When we seek an explanation we find that medical schools vastly increased the numbers of clinical professors on their staffs during this time, from about 11,000 to 78,000. This growth corresponds with the greater importance placed on practice plan income that the staff generated during this period, increasing from approximately 5 to 50 percent of the medical schools' budgets.

By the early to mid-1980s problems were becoming apparent in the favorable reimbursement environment that had been in place between private insurance plans and the federal government since the implementation of Medicare. (Although hospital inpatient admissions dropped off at the beginning of the 1980s and never recovered, the number of outpatient procedures that hospitals provided started to increase. This trend has continued right up to today.) Congress attempted several efforts to find a more economical way for the federal government to reimburse hospitals for treating Medicare patients other than its long-in-place cost-plus methodology. In 1983 Congress finally adopted the prospective payment system (PPS), predicated on diagnostic related groups (DRGs). This system stipulated in advance the amount that the federal government would pay for each principal diagnosis, irrespective of the hospital's costs. If the hospital's costs were below the designated payment level it could keep the difference; otherwise it would have to absorb the loss.

The passage of Medicare also resulted in little appreciated but important additional consequences. One was the unplanned contributions that it made to upgrade the level of hospital care provided by smaller suburban and exurban hospitals for their fast-growing populations. Another result was the explosive growth in specialists, led by the efforts of AHCs to greatly expand the number of specialty-trained physicians. Third was the growing preference of the American people to be treated close to home. In the pre–World War II era people who lived or vacationed in New England quickly learned that the New England Medical Center in Boston had established opportunities for some members of its staff to spend time at outlying hospitals interacting with local physicians. These local physicians were encouraged to refer their more complicated cases to Boston for admission and treatment. Similarly, upper-income, well-educated Atlantic coast residents between Florida and Virginia recognized that their best option was to head for Duke or Johns Hopkins University in the event of a serious medical condition. If they wintered not too distantly, they might seek admission to Vanderbilt at Nashville. Most better-educated members of higher-income groups recognized that they would be better served by turning to a major medical center for treatment of a serious illness or injury rather than seeking care at a nearby hospital. The staff of the local hospitals usually included few specialists, and these facilities were unlikely to have the latest equipment. The overall level of patient treatment most often fell well below the AHCs' centers of excellence.

Medicare and changes associated with this legislation transformed this situation, however, over the next 20 years. Millions who lived in the suburbs of large cities or in smaller outlying communities found vastly expanded local accessibility to a more sophisticated level of medical and surgical care. The sizable funds that Medicare made available for the training of specialists and subspecialists, and the avidity with which the graduates of U.S. medical schools as well as thousands of international medical graduates sought training in one or another specialty, created an explosive growth in the supply of newly trained specialists.

The parallel stimulus that Medicare offered to reimburse hospitals on a cost-plus basis allowed many smaller community hospitals to upgrade. Without this local expansion and upgrading, the growth in the numbers of new specialists certainly would have leveled off much earlier. The newly board-certified specialists would have encountered difficulty in finding suitable locations to establish practices. On the one hand the much expanded supply of specialists coincided with the accessibility of capital funding via Medicare reimbursements; on the other hand many of the relocated suburban and exurban populations exercised their preferences to be treated close to home. Together these dynamics created the preconditions for expanding more sophisticated health and hospital facilities in outlying areas.

But stresses and strains started to emerge in the early 1980s in certain hospital market areas, such as southern California. These conditions were reflected in an increasing number of excess hospital beds as well as in the growing numbers of physicians who faced varying degrees of difficulty in keeping their appointment schedules filled. Slowly but surely conditions changed as managed care companies, mostly for-profit, recognized the opportunities that these market areas with surplus beds and surplus physicians offered. This situation also worked to the advantage of the large employers who had long provided health insurance coverage for their workers and their dependents and who had begun to pay more attention to the steady rise in their health benefit premium rates. Now that the employer community wanted to slow its cost increases, managed care companies were well positioned to drive hard bargains with hospital providers facing surplus capacity and with physicians, particularly specialists, with free appointment time.

As the century drew to an end, and after two decades of a growing excess of acute care hospital beds, the hospital sector cannot be easily summarized. First, the larger community and teaching hospitals made substantial upgrades over the past three decades or longer, and they added large numbers of well-trained specialists to their staffs. They also obtained the capital required to upgrade their facilities, equipment, and support staffs to position most of these hospitals to provide quality tertiary care. A related generalization is the sizable increase in routine and sophisticated ambulatory care services that most hospitals have been able to add. This capability is important because Medicare did not cap reimbursements for ambulatory care as it did with DRGs on those for inpatient care. The best explanation for the upward trend in hospitals' net profit margins over the past 10 or more years despite an ever-reduced demand for inpatient care is the profitability of their rapidly expanding same-day surgical services. Their cost reductions may be the second explanation.

Many smaller as well as poorly located larger hospitals have been forced to merge or close during the past decade and longer, and average national occupancy rates are in the 60 percent range—and considerably lower in certain market areas. Nevertheless most hospitals have so far been able to cope with the pressures that the managed care environment has brought in its wake by cutting the number of certified beds among other operating reductions. The future is admittedly problematic, but so long as the Medicare system continues to function much as it has in the past, and assuming no radical changes occur in the private health insurance market, the U.S. hospital sector is likely to keep performing with reasonable efficiency and effectiveness. If as some believe, however, admissions continue to drop precipitously, the time is probably not that far off when significant hospital downscaling will require renewed attention and action.

Despite the forebodings of the AMA leadership in the early 1960s, the passage of Medicare did not put American medicine on the road to a socialist debacle. Rather, Medicare set the scene for a striking upgrading of the hospital care services available to the American people. At the same time liberal reimbursement policies have made it possible for American physicians, generalists, and specialists alike to enjoy an almost uninterrupted increase in their annual earnings, which only now is becoming tempered by the need to hire more staff to handle insurers and by the demands of compliance requirements to guidelines issued by managed care.

To be more thorough in our analysis, we also need to consider some of the more important intersecting trends between the Medicare-covered elderly and the nonelderly poor who qualified for government-financed medical and hospital care under Medicaid. It is hard to believe, but when Medicaid was about to be implemented in 1966 active recruitment campaigns were launched in New York City to speed enrollments through advertising in the subways as well as campaigns on the campuses of universities. In the early 1970s beneficiaries of Supplemental Security Income

(SSI) became eligible for Medicaid, and those who met Medic-aid's income requirements could be admitted for routine nursing home care, with Medicaid paying the bill. This later provision was intended to benefit the poor, but it became equally important to many middle-income people who met Medicaid's eligibility requirements by transferring their funds earlier to other members of the family or by "spending down" their assets because of an extended stay in a nursing home.

By the mid-1970s Medicaid had enrolled about 70 percent of all persons who fell below the federal poverty level. But three factors caused this relatively high enrollment percentage to drop precipitously over the next decade to an estimated 40 percent. First, cutbacks in federal support for Medicaid occurred from 1981 to 1984. Second, as a consequence of the severe recession of 1981–82 the number of poor people grew considerably. Third, the system was confronted with steeply rising medical costs, particularly hospital costs, severely straining on the budgets of many states.

In the mid-1980s Congress became concerned with the low ranking of the United States among nations on such criteria as infant mortality rates and other statistics. In response, Congress made successive groups of mothers and young children eligible for Medicaid coverage even if the family income exceeded the previously established Medicaid criteria. In 1988 Congress went further and passed the Catastrophic Amendments to Medicare to ease the difficulties that many of the elderly poor were facing in paying the deductibles and copayments required of Medicare beneficiaries. To the surprise of many, most of the 1988 statute was repealed in late 1989, largely because of the opposition of the affluent elderly who, under the new legislation, had to cover the additional costs of the 1988 amendment—amounting to as much as $1,300 of additional taxes per couple per annum. Because most of the wealthy had access to other sources to pay for the additional coverage that the 1988 legislation provided, it is not surprising that they sought to repeal the legislation. What is surprising is that they succeeded— although not entirely. Congress continued to enforce Medicaid's obligation to pay the additional costs that the poor elderly enrolled in Medicare would otherwise have to meet. In 1997 the joint beneficiaries of both Medicare and Medicaid accounted for about 6 million, or 16 percent of Medicare enrollment, and this group was responsible for $53 billion in Medicare expenses.

Having complicated the analysis by focusing on the poor elderly enrolled in both Medicare and Medicaid, we believe that it is important to step back and consider the significant differences between the Medicare reimbursement practices of the federal government and the Medicaid practices pursued by most states. Medicare paid the key providers—physicians and hospitals—an approximation of their accustomed fees and charges. This payment helped to ensure that Medicare beneficiaries would have broad access to mainstream U.S. medical care. The provider community viewed and treated this population as desirable patients. The resolution was quite different when it came to the Medicaid population, for whom state governments set the rules. Medical care for many of the poor has remained marginal. Medicaid funding is usually very tight, and about half of the eligible population loses its eligibility for Medicaid benefits every 24 months. Moreover, most U.S.-trained physicians avoid practicing in low-income neighborhoods or accepting positions at public hospitals, which provide much of the care for Medicaid enrollees. In New York State, for example, a routine Medicaid patient office visit in the 1990s commanded a fee of $13. Even before the passage of

Medicare and Medicaid the large public hospital system in New York City had to work out special affiliation contracts with several of the AHCs to provide and supervise residency staff. These staffs were heavily composed of international medical graduates, as many U.S.-trained physicians shunned such assignments.

The steady increase in the total number of the uninsured after the mid-1980s reached over 43 million in late 1998 and is still increasing. Partly as a consequence of the new federal welfare legislation passed in 1996, various subgroups of the poor, such as recent immigrants, have experienced increased difficulty in qualifying for Medicaid. These events indicate the clear contrast between the two programs: although Medicare has been a great success in providing most of the poor elderly access to mainstream ambulatory and inpatient care, Medicaid has often fallen short.

Another example further delineates this contrast. Medicare brought the elderly and selected groups of the disabled (including all who suffer from end stage renal disease, irrespective of age) into the mainstream physician and hospital treatment systems by reimbursing providers at about the same rates as patients covered by private health insurance. The financial and administrative oversight of Medicare rest solely with the federal government. In contrast, primary administrative responsibility for Medicaid devolves upon the states, which are obligated to raise between 20 and 50 percent of the costs of their Medicaid program. As a result, a significant number of the poorer states fail to cover more than a subset of their population with incomes below the federal poverty level. Moreover, the extent of coverage for an individual can vary widely between states.

The passage of the Balanced Budget Act of 1997 sets the stage for radical changes in Medicare in the coming years, although relatively few changes have been introduced to date. In the early 1970s Congress broadened Medicare coverage to two groups of patients below the age of 65: those who suffered from End Stage Renal Disease and previously active members of the workforce who were below the age of 65 and who were on Social Security Disability Income. Other than these two exceptions, Congress held the line on Medicare eligibility.

Starting in the early 1980s, however, Congress introduced innovations that affected the benefit side of the Medicare equation. First was the opportunity for risk-based HMOs to enroll Medicare beneficiaries and make payments based on 95 percent of the costs of providing care in a given area for the predominantly Medicare population enrolled in fee-for-service coverage. Because of the economies that the prepayment plans were able to achieve as a result of favorable self-selection, Medicare beneficiaries often received additional benefits. What is more, because of the way in which the federal government had set its risk-based reimbursement rate, it paid only about 5 percent more than the outlays that Medicare would have had to make had the enrollees remained in the dominant fee-for-service arrangement. The second significant change on the Medicare benefit side was an outgrowth of the Medicare Catastrophic Amendments Act of 1988, most provisions of which, as already mentioned were rescinded the following year. But the 1988 provision establishing joint Medicare–Medicaid coverage for the elderly who were below the federal poverty level was not canceled, and so the poor elderly could continue to rely on Medicaid to pay a range of collateral costs. These include the first day's hospitalization, the 20 percent copayment for physician services, and the costs of outpatient drugs.

Also occurring in the late 1980s were a rapid increase in the number of persons served, the number of visits, and the total charges by Medicare Home Health services. The number of people served rose from 1.6 million in 1988 to 3.5 million in 1995. The number of visits increased during the same period from 38 million to 249 million. Total charges for the much increased number of visits exploded to $21.6 billion, up from $2.5 billion 7 years earlier (*Health Care Financing Review, Medicare and Medicaid Statistical Supplement,* 1997, p. 126).

In passing the Balanced Budget Act of 1997, Congress set the stage for the first large-scale, radical restructuring of the Medicare statute since its original passage. It is more apposite to explore some of the emerging consequences of this radical innovation in the next chapter. We will review these changes within the context of the rapid growth of managed care enrollments. This imminent restructuring will provide the new framework for altering the delivery of medical care services to the Medicare and Medicaid populations with the intention of providing service along the same lines as the privately insured.

3
Changes in the Physician Supply

When we look back at the twentieth century, we can clearly identify the importance of physician supply issues in the evolution of U.S. health care policy. From 1900 until the end of World War II, members and leaders of the AMA largely decided most questions affecting the numbers and characteristics of students who were admitted to and graduated from U.S. medical schools. The AMA and its state affiliates, working closely with the leadership of the nation's medical schools, operated under broad grants of authority and autonomy from state legislatures that held formal control over the licensing of medical practitioners. In cooperation with other medical groups such as the early specialist societies, the AMA was able to control the numbers of students entering the medical profession. Between the early 1930s and the end of World War II, the AMA kept the number of new, licensed practitioners under tight control. During this time, the only other major parties of interest concerning the nation's physician supply were some of the leading philanthropies, notably Carnegie and Rockefeller. Both of these foundations devoted considerable attention and resources toward raising the educational and professional standards of the successive cohorts of medical students.

The large-scale relocation of many rural populations, both intra- and interstate, and the rising levels of employment and income helped to add the expansion of physician supply to the nation's health agenda. As we noted earlier, however, conditions were changing: higher living standards prevailed, large geographical movements affected many Americans, and curative medicine had demonstrated new efficacy. Not surprisingly, pressure began to build as early as 1948 for the federal government to seek funding from Congress to expand the physician supply. But in the face of AMA opposition, Congress failed to respond.

Pressure continued to mount, however, and in his second administration President Dwight D. Eisenhower appointed three high-level committees to assess the need for special efforts. But he did not accept their strong recommendations favoring federal action toward expanding the supply of physicians. Not until 1963, when the AMA concentrated its lobbying strength against Medicare, was Congress able to act by initiating liberal financing of medical and other health professional schools. This funding continued until 1976, when Congress decided that the physician shortage had finally ended. During this expansion, the number of medical school graduates doubled from around 7,500 to 15,000 annually, reaching a peak of about 16,300 in the early 1980s.

Two legislative actions of Congress in 1964 and 1965 also had long-term impact on the future supply of physicians: the Civil Rights Act and the revision of the long-in-place immigration and naturalization statutes. In 1964, Congress amended and passed the civil rights bill that President John F. Kennedy had submitted shortly before his assassination. The Johnson administration subsequently proposed to broaden the bill to prohibit discrimination in employment, but powerful southerners in Congress opposed to the bill slowed its progress. At the suggestion of several of his advisers, Senator Joseph Clark of Pennsylvania, one of the leaders in the effort for a broadened statute, extended the antidiscrimination provision from race to include gender to garner additional support for the bill's passage. The bill ultimately passed with multiple consequences for altering the size and composition of the U.S. physician supply.

The bill's biggest impact was on the growth in the number of woman physicians. In the 1960s, the United States had the smallest representation of women physicians (fewer than 1 in 10) among the advanced nations, Spain alone excepted. In the succeeding decades the proportion of women entering U.S. medical schools increased more than fivefold. As the century neared its end, women accounted for over 40 percent of current graduates.

In the early 1970s, Eli Ginzberg attended a meeting of the the Association of American Medical Colleges, where the theme was the expansion in the supply of women physicians. Because the Civil Rights Act of 1964 prohibited discrimination based on either race or gender, he remarked at the meeting, many more women inevitably would be accepted into medical school, because they represented the largest untapped pool of well-qualified candidates. Indeed, the gains in the number and proportion of African American (and Hispanic) enrollees would be much more constrained given the limited numbers of qualified applicants. Nonetheless, their numbers increased as well, about threefold, although from a very low level.

In 1965, Congress decided to revise its highly restrictive immigration and naturalization laws and regulations that had been

in place since the early 1920s. The revision was designed to enlarge the total annual inflow and to reverse the prior heavy discrimination in favor of immigrants from western and northern
Europe. The reform legislation succeeded: Senator Edward Kennedy of Massachusetts and other sponsors pointed out years later
that they had not anticipated the three- to fourfold increase in the
annual number of new arrivals—the result of the revised quotas.
As part of this reform Congress did not intend to open wide
the gates to graduates of foreign medical schools (IMGs) to do
their residency training in the United States, but this is exactly
what happened. Many of these graduates subsequently altered
their student visas to enable them to remain in the country and
practice. This group currently accounts for about 175,000 out of
the total national pool of 730,000 physicians. Many IMGs, upon
completion of their residency, were ready to accept positions that
American graduates avoided. The needs of many communities
for improved access to physicians were much ameliorated by this
action. In turn, the willingness of these graduates to start practices
in underserved communities helped to deflect potential criticism
against the established medical leadership for not having provided
effective remedies.

The linkages between Congressional actions on these fronts—
to finance medical education, to weaken discrimination in employment, and to revise the immigration and naturalization statutes—
and their impact on the future of the AHCs and medical care for
the American people still remain to be delineated.

The Medicare and Medicaid statutes were implemented July 1,
1966. The impact of these laws on the physician supply raises
several questions: How were the number and the types of AHC-
trained physicians affected? What changed at the principal teach-

ing hospitals? How did the reimbursement policies of the programs affect the long-term reorientation of the AHCs? What were their consequences on the future incomes and practice locations of physicians? As part of this Medicare era, we will also describe the further impacts on the physician supply following the rapid growth of managed care plans in the late 1980s- and early 1990s. We will also consider the uncertain physician policy outlook as the new century begins.

The Medicare statute, and to a lesser extent Medicaid, affected the future physician supply in many dimensions—in numbers, specialization, practice locations, and incomes. It also had a major impact on the teaching hospitals involved in the education and training of students and residents. And it accelerated the provision of increasingly sophisticated care that physicians provided to their more seriously ill and injured patients, another key factor influencing the physician supply.

To begin with, Medicare provided multiple sources of graduate medical education (GME) funding to the AHCs and other teaching hospitals for the direct and indirect expenditures associated with their sponsorship of residency training programs. This amounted to a sizable new source of funding; even though Medicare's GME dollars related only to the proportion of Medicare patients cared for, this figure has grown to over $6 billion annually. Consequently, residents' stipends were raised to at least a maintenance level of income, approximately $30,000 to $40,000 annually—considerably more than they had been able to earn before Medicare. Increased stipends made it easier for the residents to pursue specialty and subspecialty training.

The GME funding and, even more important, the liberal reimbursement for Medicare inpatient care encouraged many of the country's leading AHCs to offer their key faculty members full-time contracts. This development allowed these individuals to become more actively engaged in the three functions of the typical AHC: education, research, and patient care. With new and enlarged funding, the AHCs could support a much greater number of residents and fellows, who, in turn, were able to oversee the routine care of many if not most hospitalized patients. Hence, senior clinicians were able to diagnose and treat a larger number of insured patients—a group that contributed directly and indirectly both to their earnings and to the revenue of the AHCs.

The funds available to the AHCs also increased in other ways following the introduction of Medicare. These additional funding sources derived more or less directly from GME, the single largest source of which resulted from the conversion of many former charity and part-pay patients into Medicare reimbursed patients. Under Medicare, hospitals were paid based on their costs for patient treatment and also for the use of their capital. By the late 1980s, hospitals that cared for large numbers of the poor also became eligible to receive "disproportionate share payments" via Medicare and Medicaid. These funds currently amount to between $15 and $20 billion annually.

By the early 1980s the large research-oriented AHCs had taken the lead in developing a new self-financing mechanism that provided additional funding for their expanding and costly innovations. They appointed large numbers of full-time clinical professors who would earn their salaries and benefits by treating private patients. At the same time these professors would, on average, contribute 10–15 percent of their salaries to the dean's fund and/or to their department's budget.

The AHCs trained ever larger numbers of residents in specialty and subspecialty areas. In part this was because the faculty recognized the benefit of a large pool of low-cost patient care activities in their assistants. But the question then arose, how would this rapidly growing specialist group be able to start a practice once the physicians had finished serving their apprenticeship? The changing conditions we have described above largely answer this question. Many affluent families had relocated to the suburbs and preferred to obtain their medical care close to home. With the liberal operating and capital funding provided by Medicare, many smaller suburban community hospitals were able to transform themselves into tertiary care institutions by appointing many of these young board-certified specialists to their expanding staffs. However, with this solution, as former Harvard Medical School dean Robert Ebert noted, the AHCs were creating their future competitors. This potential competition did not seem to concern the leading AHCs until the 1980s and 1990s, during which time admissions for inpatient hospital care declined significantly. But even more troubling was the rapid growth of managed care, which brought with it restrictions in patient self-referrals to specialists, further reducing admissions for inpatient care. Managed care plans also shortened lengths of stay for those admitted. The intensified efforts of managed care administrators to seek out lower-cost institutions if and when inpatient hospital care had to be authorized for their enrollees further raised the competitive stakes.

Congress early questioned the effect of its two principal interventions, targeted funding for expanding the capacity of the nation's medical schools and the multiple spending streams from Medicare. Were they an adequate response to the needs of the American people for broader access to physicians? Members of Congress were being repeatedly apprised by their constituents in underserved urban and rural areas of the serious difficulty they had in accessing physicians. Hence, in passing legislation creating the National Health Services Corps in 1970, Congress intervened anew. This legislation was intended to improve the distribution of the existing supply of physicians to ensure some relief for areas that continued to be underserved. It provided for educational debt cancellation and income bonuses for physicians who would accept one-year or longer assignments in underserved areas. At its peak in the late 1970s and early 1980s, the program had assigned about 3,500 physicians to shortage areas. The program also provided additional numbers of mid-level health care workers, particularly nurses.

But in the early 1980s, the Reagan administration acted to curtail the program, saying that the program had failed to improve significantly the number of physicians available to diagnose and treat underserved populations. Later, both the Bush and Clinton administrations sought and received additional new funding from Congress to revive the earlier, much shrunken effort. However, the funding never reached the scale and scope that would have been required to compensate for market shortfalls in distributing the physician supply more equitably among high- and low-income locations.

In 1971, the year following the passage of the national health service legislation, Congress undertook a related initiative to mitigate the maldistribution problem. Physician advocates in the agricultural areas of the Midwest had earlier concluded that many small and medium-sized communities had need for more general practitioners. Responding to this critique, Congress offered to fund family practice residencies to increase the number of primary care physicians.

In retrospect, we can venture several generalizations about this federal initiative. Indeed, a considerable number of AHCs and other teaching hospitals responded to the congressional offer of funding for family practice residencies. But it is noteworthy that the leading research-oriented AHCs initially were conspicuously absent among the applicants. Not until the early 1990s did the AHCs seek to respond to the strengthening market for family physicians, general internists, and general pediatricians, many of whom the growing managed care system employed as gatekeepers.

In the two decades following the new federal support, and notwithstanding the continuing efforts of the Robert Wood Johnson Foundation to encourage the output of primary care practitioners, the data show a striking and steady decline in the number of residents training for a career in primary care. Only in the 1990s do the data point to a pronounced if belated shift in favor of primary care training. Between 1993 and 1997 the number of medical school graduates selecting a primary care specialty for their residency training doubled in the fields of family practice, general internal medicine, and pediatrics.

A number of factors influence the distribution of physicians between primary care and specialty and subspecialty training. The cutting edge of medical knowledge and treatment was definitely linked with the advances in specialty care, which was the focus of the nation's leading biomedical research centers. The reward structure, academic distinction, and monetary income were all heavily tilted in the direction of the specialties. On average, specialists earn twice that of primary care physicians, and a minority of specialists are able to earn $500,000 or more per annum.

Some other conditions also bear on the tensions between the two types of practice—generalist and specialist. Many of the new medical schools established after 1963 (assisted by newly available federal funds) were relatively small schools located in underserved, low-density areas that were in need of attracting more general practitioners. But because the majority of the U.S. population lives in metropolitan areas (4 out of 5 by the late 1990s), many medical students hesitated to prepare themselves for a professional future that would require them and their families to live in a community of 25,000. Their hesitancy was that much greater if they had grown up in a large metropolitan area and had attended a medical school and pursued residency training at a large AHC located in a major urban center.

One additional observation: with much of the demand for physicians' services centered among the elderly, many with chronic conditions, a significant part of many specialists' practices has been to serve as the principal physician for patients who have one or more chronic diseases. It is unclear whether it makes any sense for the nation, having produced a more than adequate supply of many types of specialists, to attempt to redirect patients toward generalists. This concern is particularly critical given the fact that the majority of Americans live in a metropolitan area where they have ready access a range of specialists who can meet the needs of different patients as well as serve as their primary care physician.

These two legislative interventions of Congress in 1970 and 1971 more or less ended the direct activist role of the federal government in seeking to improve access for underserved groups by restructuring the physician supply. But there was a more indirect exception for which we need to refer again to our discussion of the international medical graduates. As more and more IMGs completed their residency training, a significant number of them were willing, at least for a limited number of years, to start practice in an underserved area.

Although definitive data are hard to come by, the 175,000 IMGs who are currently practicing in the United States fill a disproportionate number of the conventionally less attractive positions. They provide large amounts of primary care services for one or more of the growing immigrant groups living in large cities, from Mexican border cities in Texas to Los Angeles, Chicago, New York, and Philadelphia. These graduates also account for many physicians attached to the staffs of public institutions such as state mental hospitals, prisons, and publicly financed acute and long-term care facilities. In addition, many have relocated for a number of years in low-income, low-density rural areas. Some decide to remain permanently after having been exposed to their practice environment and having found it to be to their liking.

The generally favorable practice environment for new physicians during the past third of the century, especially for those who were willing to relocate to outlying locations and/or accept institutional appointments, ensured that most IMGs who desired to remain in the United States to practice had the opportunity to do so. It was not until the early to mid-1990s that a number of professional groups representing mainstream medical organizations began to raise serious questions about the future absorption rate of this group of physicians.

For twenty years or more after the implementation of Medicare, the AHCs and the medical profession at large enjoyed an upbeat professional environment in most U.S. regions. The profession was characterized by both high prestige and high earnings. By 1976 Congress decided that it had succeeded in the special effort that it had launched in 1963 to provide substantial federal financing to expand the supply of physicians and other health care personnel and terminated its subsidization now that the shortages had been eliminated.

In reaching this decision, Congress also provided for the appointment of a committee — the Graduate Medical Education National Advisory Committee (GMENAC). This committee was charged with assessing the longer-term outlook for the number and types of physicians that should be trained so that the American people could be assured that they had ready access to both generalists and specialists. Reporting in 1980 and 1981, the committee concluded that the United States confronted a large prospective surplus of physicians amounting to about 70,000 in 1990 and close to 145,000 at century's end. This forecast attracted little attention in the midst of the economic recession that accompanied Ronald Reagan's entrance into the White House. The committee's findings also left the medical schools, the specialty societies, and practicing physicians unimpressed. The environments in which physicians were operating and their appointment schedules and annual earnings provided little support for these harsh forecasts in the predominantly fee-for-service environment; at the time, each person entering the practice of medicine was more or less assured of adding $250,000 annually to health care costs and taking home, on average, about 40 percent of that sum.

The disregard of the committee's reports by most leaders and members of the AMA and the specialty societies in the early 1980s can best be appreciated by reviewing the forces that came to dominate the health care marketplace after the passage of Medicare and Medicaid. For the next fifteen years throughout the United States, and for another decade in many regions within the nation, the different parts of the health care system became disconnected.

Patients seeking medical care, physicians delivering medical care, and employers or government paying for medical care were not in balanced economic relationships. Not until the early to mid-1980s did connections between demand for health care services and a consideration of their costs start to reemerge slowly. This new trend was made possible at least in part by the growing amount of excess capacity in hospital facilities and the free appointment time in the schedules of many specialists in vulnerable health care market areas.

Several observations are pertinent regarding the impact of these and related developments on the physician supply and on the financing of the multiple missions of the leading AHCs: for the first time since the Great Depression, selected physicians, especially among subspecialists, faced a falloff in the demand for their services. Some professionals even contemplated moving to another state to avoid suffering significant reductions in their earnings. The new medical marketplace also increased the demand for primary care physicians, because, as we mentioned above, managed care companies eagerly sought to employ them as gatekeepers. The companies expected that this strategy would help reduce enrollees' indiscriminate use of specialists as well as attempts to seek unnecessary referrals for inpatient hospital care. With the rapid growth in managed care enrollments and ever tighter controls by managed care plans over the choices that patients were free to make, the average annual earnings of physicians in 1994 showed a decline—the first since the introduction of Medicare and Medicaid, in fact since the end of World War II.

The related question that we need to explore at least briefly is, what impact did the increasingly tumultuous market changes of the 1980s and 1990s have on the leading AHCs? Without ascribing any specific significance to their ordering, the following three developments warrant attention. First, there were very few medical school closures: Oral Roberts in Tulsa ceased operations in 1990, and the Medical College of Pennsylvania merged with Hahnemann University in Philadelphia in 1995. At the beginning of 1998 several additional merger discussions were under way but had not yet been finalized when this book went into publication.

Second, selected reductions have occurred in the numbers of residents applying for, and accepted into, subspecialty residency training programs. At the same time there has been a correspondingly large increase in the numbers of students and residents electing to major in a primary care specialty. And many of the research-oriented AHCs that earlier had shunned sponsoring family care residencies have rethought their early decision and have since added such programs.

The third development reflects a growing destabilization of the acute care sector of the U. S. health care marketplace since the mid- to late 1980s. Yet most of the research-oriented AHCs have generated sufficient additional revenues from their practice plans to compensate for the reduced flows of patients referred by managed care plans and the corresponding reductions in customary charges. In addition, residents completing their training in selected specialties, from pathology and anesthesiology to ophthalmology and cardiology, have encountered increasing difficulties in entering practices with a favorable outlook for future growth. Awareness of the reality of these markets has tended to steer young physicians away from these specialties.

The predominantly privately insured population has been rapidly transferred into managed care plans, and more publicly insured persons likely will also enroll voluntarily or under compulsion. New projections examine the implications that such rapid growth will have on the future requirements for physician supply numbers overall as well as the desirable ratio of primary care physicians to specialists and subspecialists.

Jonathan Wiener at Johns Hopkins University and David Kindig of the University of Wisconsin have conducted independent studies and have made two of the more carefully designed and executed projections. The conclusions they reach are similar and point to an excess supply of approximately 150,000 physicians. This calculation reflects a number of factors. Their studies expect reduced referral rates to specialists, fewer admissions to acute care hospitals, more attention to preventive services, and the greater deployment of midlevel personnel in the provision of medical services to managed care enrollees. But the question that needs to be asked and at least provisionally answered is the extent to which the current health care marketplace provides even partial confirmation of this conclusion.

Several recent developments point to increasing disquietude about the growing size of physician supply. Three prestigious groups of medical leaders—the AAMC, the AMA, and COGME (the congressionally appointed council to advise the federal legislators on future trends in the physician supply) have made joint recommendations to Congress. They propose that Congress reduce the number of IMG admissions to the United States and into residency programs to no more than 10 percent (approximately 1,600) of the number of annual graduates of U.S. medical schools. This plan is in sharp contrast to recent numbers of IMG entrants into residency training, which have totaled over three times this recommended quota.

The proposal to cut back and limit future numbers of IMGs

admitted into the country and into residency training programs is reinforced by a growing position among many within the medical educational leadership. Their concern is that the time may not be that far off when U. S. medical schools and residency programs will have to address the issue of large reductions in numbers accepted. In their view it would be totally inappropriate to recommend the cutback and possible closure of selected U.S. medical schools in the face of continuing unrestricted inflow of IMGs.

Coincidentally, the Pew Health Professions Commission, under the chairmanship of former governor Richard Lamm of Colorado, publicly recommended in 1995 that by 2005 the United States should take action to reduce its graduating medical school class from the current 16,000 figure to around 13,500. The commission further recommended that by that same date 25 percent of the currently 124 operating allopathic medical schools be closed. But as of 2000, the Pew commission recommendation has elicited relatively little attention and even less action.

In a separate but related development, the Health Care Financing Administration (HCFA) launched a demonstration program in 1997 with selected major AHCs and teaching hospitals in New York State and negotiated prospective agreements with selected other states. The pilot program attempted to provide a financial cushion for sponsoring institutions that agree to cut back their residency training programs over a five-year period, representing the first policy initiative focused on constraining the future number of physicians. But reports as of the end of 1999 indicate that a majority of the participating AHCs have withdrawn from the demonstration.

Before ending this chapter on physician supply policy, we should consider a number of related health workforce issues during the past third of a century. These are issues that to various degrees grow out of our earlier focus on the education and training of medical students and residents in allopathic schools, the mainstream institutions of U.S. medicine.

In the past three decades, schools of osteopathy whose graduates had not previously been recognized by the dominant allopathic sector were able to work out new arrangements. Their graduates were increasingly admitted into residency programs and obtained staff positions in hospitals that belonged to the mainstream allopathic tradition. In 1999, 19 schools of osteopathy were in operation with a total enrollment of just under 9,000. The 1997 graduating class numbered 2,020, or roughly 11 percent of the number of graduates of all medical schools, allopathic and osteopathic, in that year.

We should also note the explosive growth since the early 1960s in the health sector workforce. Today this number approximates 11.5 million, or slightly less than 1 out of every 10 employed persons in the United States. Nursing is the single largest component, representing different levels of educational background and training, from the completion of a two-year course in a community college to a baccalaureate, master's, or doctor's degree. Most state medical societies (that is, physicians) have used their political influence with their respective legislatures to restrict the scope of practice by nurses, including prohibiting them from writing prescriptions. But under pressure from underserved populations, government health officials, and, more recently, managed care plans, the responsibilities of nurses with advanced training have broadened. In many cases nurses can substitute for primary care physicians, and in some instances they have won the right to admit patients to community and teaching hospitals.

Changes in the Physician Supply

Registered nurses outnumber physicians by a ratio of more than 3 to 1. Along with the current trend of lowering and removing the long-established restrictions on the scope of practice for nurses with graduate training, payers for health care are looking for new ways to economize in the delivery of health care services, and many groups of patients express a preference for being treated by nurses. In light of these factors, further discussions and actions affecting the future supply of physicians will have to consider current and potential future changes in the scope of practice of both physicians and nurses.

Clearly, the discussion of the expanding as well as the changing character of the physician supply in the United States involves many factors, particularly since the passage of Medicare. To recapitulate some of the important points we have covered:

- The introduction and maintenance of large-scale federal funding for the enlargement of existing medical schools and the establishment of approximately 40 new medical schools resulted in a doubling in the annual output of U.S. medical schools from around 8,000 to more than 16,000 over a thirteen-year period.
- The 1965 and later revisions of the immigration and naturalization statutes enabled large numbers of IMGs to come to the United States for residency training and, if they so desired, to remain here to practice. They account today for approximately 1 out of every 4 physicians in active practice.
- Concerned parties have almost completely disregarded the four-year, in-depth study by the congressionally appointed medical education advisory committee. The committee's 1980–81 findings reported that the country faced large prospective surpluses of physicians in 1990 and 2000.

- The trend in physician earnings, with the exception of 1994, continues upward despite the greatly increased number of physicians who are in practice and large number of insured patients now enrolled in managed care plans, which seek to exercise closer control over their enrollees' open-ended use of physician services. The leading research-oriented AHCs continued to focus on the training of specialists and subspecialists until very recently when first-year residents began a strong shift toward selecting primary care residencies. Whether they will seek to enter practice or pursue further residency training in a specialty upon completion of their initial board certification remains to be seen, however. Also unclear is the extent to which large numbers of patients will be satisfied to receive their treatment from primary care physicians over the long term.
- The well-planned and executed research studies in the 1990s concluded that, with the major shift of the U.S. public into a managed care plan, the total physician supply requirements should decline by around 25 percent from the earlier, predominantly fee-for-service system. As yet there is little support for this conclusion other than growing evidence that entrants into selected specialties and subspecialties are encountering difficulties in locating attractive practice opportunities and that the earnings of those in selected specialties have declined.
- The only stirrings in the policy arena to affect the future size of the physician supply have been the combined recommendations of the AAMC, the AMA, and COGME to Congress to cut back radically on the number of IMGs authorized to enter the United States to pursue residency training. A related development has been the failing demonstration launched by HCFA with the AHCs and teaching hospitals in New York State. The

plan provided for HCFA to cushion the revenue reductions over a five-year period for hospitals that agree to cut back on the number of residents that they accept into their training programs, but the demonstration has run into serious trouble.

• Although the Pew Health Professions Commission report of 1995 recommended cutbacks in U.S. medical school graduates from over 16,000 annually to around 13,000 by 2005, resulting in the closure of 25 percent of the 124 AHCs currently in operation, the recommendation has elicited little attention and less follow-up.

With this review to guide us, we can make the following two assessments. First, so long as the total annual expenditures for the health care sector are on a steep upward curve, from $1 trillion in annual outlays in 1996 to $2 trillion by 2007, the present and prospective supply of physicians should be able to find reasonable opportunities to practice and to earn a satisfactory income. Second, given the continuation of current spending conditions, effective controls will not likely be introduced in the near future to restrict the supply of physicians. The possible exception is a policy change to reduce the number of IMGs permitted to immigrate, enter residency training, and remain in this country to practice. This state of nonaction could change if and when the federal and state governments together with the nonprofit and for-profit sectors enter into a joint planning effort to place some broad limits on the annual rate of new spending for health care. Simultaneously the issue of the future supply of physicians would have to appear on the national policy agenda for specific analysis, discussion, and action.

4
Challenging the AHCs to Change

American medicine won the acclaim of most informed observers of the post–World War II era for its steady advances in biomedical research and in the delivery of high-tech medical treatment. A number of dissenters, however, have questioned whether the accomplishments warranted such unqualified praise. Experts in social medicine in Great Britain, for example, have pointed out that the greatest gains in reduced morbidity and lengthened life expectancy were more indicative of changes in the socioeconomic environment than advances in curative medicine. These researchers demonstrated that mortality rates among the various classes remained the same during the three decades that the British National Health Service had been operational. Throughout the years 1950 to 1980, those in the lowest ranks of the civil service continued to have a noticeably shorter life span than those in the higher ranks.

In the early 1970s Marc LaLonde, minister of health in the Canadian federal government, advanced the idea that the government should make a radical shift in its health care programs and expenditures by focusing on public health and prevention to improve the health status of its citizens. At that time the government supported broadened access to treatment and more effective cures of diseases that compel individual patients to seek treatment from physicians and hospitals. Although LaLonde's proposal attracted considerable attention, its longer-term impact on Canadian medicine resulted in an emphasis on the importance of periodic health examinations and the on role of personal behavior in contributing to overall health. But Canada's physicians continued to focus energy on meeting the challenges of curative medicine.

The United States has been the recognized leader of clinical medicine after World War II, as the country's leading research universities and AHCs captured a disproportionate share of Nobel prizes for medicine. The prevailing professional consensus at home and overseas was that the leading AHCs were at the forefront of providing the most sophisticated medical and surgical treatment. But it would be a mistake to assume that admiration and approval in the United States was universal. A few dissenters could be identified, among them was Kerr White of Johns Hopkins University. White, a physician with strong training in public health, found many weaknesses in the organization and management of the U.S. health care system. He took issue with its preoccupation with the treatment and cure of disease rather than the need to address a broader concern—improving the health status of the population at large and its handicapped subgroups, such as racial minorities, the poor, and the less educated.

By the mid-1980s others began voicing related concerns, criticisms, and challenges regarding the emphasis on further development of high-tech medicine to reduce illness and extend the healthy life span of Americans. Much of this concern was based on the rapid increases in federal and total national expenditures for health care. A few academic economists, including Victor Fuchs of Stanford University, looked more closely at the annual dollar costs of the U.S. health care sector and the returns that individuals and the nation at large were receiving from the steeply increasing annual health care expenditures. The explosive advance of the AIDS epidemic by the mid-1980s, resulting in the premature death of tens of thousands of Americans, was a potent wake-up call. Despite its many achievements, U.S. medicine confronted increasingly serious challenges of knowledge, care, cure, and cost.

The mid-1980s presented one further challenge to American medicine. The country now faced the gap between the medical profession's contribution to the improved health and functioning of the poor and the marginal access to health care for these millions of low-income urban and rural residents. Not only did this dilemma reflect a failure to introduce a system of universal health insurance coverage for Americans, but it also reflected the shortcomings of Medicaid. Further, the situation highlighted the anomaly within the urban AHCs, home to most of the nation's medical leaders, which continued to implement their priorities with little or no interest in or concern for the unmet health care needs of the urban poor, many of whom lived nearby.

In 1986 two of the nation's leading philanthropic foundations, Rockefeller and the Pew Charitable Trusts, decided to encourage the AHCs to modify the curriculum of their medical schools. They believed that as a first step the curriculum should provide more instruction for students in epidemiology, population medicine, and public health. This approach would be in contrast to the AHCs' almost exclusive preoccupation with a patho-physiological approach to the study and treatment of disease. Accordingly, the foundations launched a liberally financed effort called the Health of the Public (HOP) program, issuing a call for proposals that was answered by 89 medical schools, representing about 7 out of 10 of the nation's allopathic schools.

The foundations decided to fund six proposals with a wide range of objectives and goals. Tufts University in Boston planned to offer a joint program in medicine and public health. Columbia University in New York proposed a program for addressing ways to provide new, improved, and expanded health care services for low-income women and children living in its adjoining low-income neighborhood. Johns Hopkins used its grant money to speed the development of its Welch Center for Prevention, Epidemiology, and Clinical Research, which became a leading epidemiological research center. It also became recognized for training investigators and strengthening academic offerings not only in the medical school but in its other health care programs as well. The University of North Carolina built interdisciplinary community-AHC partnerships to improve the access of low-income rural populations to improved medical care, while providing experience for residents to practice among the rural poor. A diverse group of UNC administrators, medical faculty, students, and staff, as well as representatives from community-based agencies, were involved in the planning and implementation of the program. The University of Washington in Seattle used its grant to create local and statewide consortia to facilitate closer collaboration among academic health centers, providers, purchasers, and government agencies with the overall goal of improving outcomes by collecting data from these providers to identify potential changes in practice. The sixth recipient was the University of New Mexico at Albuquerque. New Mexico is a very large state that has large numbers of Native Americans, Mexican Americans, and many other low-income groups living in sparsely settled areas. The grants came at a time when the faculty, which had a strong interest in preventive medicine, was in an early stage of curriculum development. The medical school used its new grant money to develop a number of programmatic innovations, including assignments of juniors and seniors to preceptor physicians in small, outlying towns. The medical students would relocate in one of these towns for a month, or even longer, not only to observe but also to participate in providing care to low-income patients.

The Pew Charitable Trusts was pleased with the number and quality of the responses to its first request for proposals. Hence in 1990, in partnership with the Robert Wood Johnson Foundation, the foundation sent out a second request. In this second round, the number of participating medical schools that received awards increased to 19. A final round of grants in 1992 raised the number of grantees to 33, with several more medical schools in affiliation but without financial support. To place this last figure in context, compare the initial solicitation, for which 70 percent of all U.S. allopathic schools submitted letters of intent, with the last award cycle, in which one quarter of the nation's medical schools received grants. Special notice needs to be given to the success of the HOP program at Chicago's Rush Medical College. Rush implemented its extensive program enthusiastically under a philosophy of demand-side learning whereby medical students were unleashed into community organizations with a problem-based orientation and served under good faculty supervision. The fact that 50 percent of Rush's graduates chose primary medicine could be attributed in great part to this program's success.

The HOP programs raise a host of critical questions: What were the three foundation sponsors trying to achieve by their grants, which totaled about $18 million from 1986 to 1996? (A final modest transition grant from the Pew Charitable Trusts enabled the interested participants to help make the transition on the termination of the HOP grant.) What are the major accomplishments of the HOP effort? What conclusions can we draw regarding the dominant forces behind the participating AHCs that limited and constrained the impact of HOP programs within both the AHC and the community? Finally, what are the broader insights that have implications for future changes in the curriculum and programming of the AHCs resulting from this foundation effort?

As stated earlier, the primary objective of the HOP program was to introduce a counterweight to U.S. medical schools' almost total preoccupation with the improved clinical treatment of disease. The foundations wished to incorporate into the curriculum at U.S. medical schools a broader appreciation that disease prevention and the prolongation of healthy years of life required an expanded focus on epidemiology, population-based medicine, and behavioral transformations. The program emphasized not only individuals but also smaller or larger groups that were encountering excessive morbidity and premature mortality. To bring about this considerable shift in faculty orientation and performance, the sponsoring foundations left it to the individual AHCs to outline the initiatives they might plan and carry through if awarded a grant.

Although curriculum reform in the medical school was a priority, program officials quickly recognized that additional gains could result if students pursuing allied disciplines such as nursing or public health were educated and trained in the same classes with medical students. In May 1992, the leaders of the curriculum reform movement issued a new mission statement in a special communication to the *Journal of the American Medical Association* (*JAMA*) titled "Health of the Public: The Academic Response." The article outlined the following propositions:

Achieving Change Within the Academic Health Center:
Objective 1—Provide basic competence in population-based subjects to all health professional students
Objective 2—Provide enhanced population-based education for selected students
Objective 3—Include clinical prevention knowledge and skill building activities at all levels of health professional education
Objective 4—Conduct substantive scholarly research in subjects related to population medicine.

By 1992 the program had extended its focus and research beyond curriculum reforms in the AHCs and outlined three additional objectives under the rubric of Achieving Change in an Academic Health Center's Role in the Community.

Objective 5—Assume institutional responsibility for maximizing the health of a defined population within available resources
Objective 6—Involve the academic health center in decision making about the development and deployment of health resources
Objective 7—Involve the academic health center in the social-political process as an advocate of the health of the public.

We have reviewed the available articles and reports since the HOP program began, and we have studied a review of the program done in late 1995 by Dr. Norman Edelman of the Robert Wood Johnson School of Medicine. We also attended the two concluding conferences sponsored by the HOP program in the spring and fall of 1996 in Boston and Philadelphia, respectively. Members of the Eisenhower Center staff have augmented our research with on-site visits to participating AHCs in Boston, New York, Philadelphia, Baltimore, Chicago, San Antonio, Albuquerque, and Los Angeles. As a result of our investigation we offer the following admittedly limited evaluation:

- The foundations' initiative succeeded in encouraging the participating AHCs to establish new and/or broadened curriculum offerings directed toward population and social medicine. At many AHCs, medical students were joined by nursing, public health, and other health services students in conjoint instruction.
- A smaller number of participating institutions introduced or expanded "enhanced population-based education for selected students."
- Relatively few AHCs responded to the two remaining objectives for curriculum reform: (1) clinical prevention knowledge and skill-building activities at all levels of health professional education, and (2) substantive scholarly research in subjects related to population medicine.

The second principal group of objectives for changing the AHC's community role sought to involve the AHC in both decision-making connected with the development and deployment of health resources and, the social/political process as a public health advocate. Although the HOP program demonstrated success in undertaking programs aimed at responding to selected health needs of the AHCs' immediate communities, it was less successful in achieving the second objective. Despite their active involvement in the HOP program, the AHCs seldom followed the suggestion that they "must define the health status and needs of a defined population of relevance and importance to the academic centers." Most AHCs were able to identify, initiate, or expand—usually in partnership with local groups—desirable preventive and other primary care services for smaller or larger subsets of the neighborhood uninsured. These services included improved immunization for preschoolers and medical services for the drug addicted and the homeless. Also implemented were support services for the infirm elderly. Many of the services were provided by students studying medical, nursing, and other health professions who were strongly motivated to improve the health status of their severely disadvantaged neighbors.

The foundations' ten-year effort to shift concentration to a population-based, preventive, social orientation was only modestly successful. Most of the gains occurred in the broadening of the medical school curriculum and the increased attention given to the unmet health care needs of the neighboring poor. However, the foundations' effort also resulted in some unanticipated dividends, including the identification and the cooperation among committed but hitherto largely isolated faculty members. They were able to meet regularly and share their experiences and aspirations for more responsible and responsive AHC efforts to improve the medical school curriculum and to focus more resources on improving the health status of their low-income neighbors.

One might argue that the HOP program achieved only modest success in shifting the balance in AHCs away from curative medicine or in making significant changes in the health care services available to their low-income neighbors. Nevertheless, the foundation support cycle represented a major challenge to the AHCs from inside the profession directed at their goals, objectives, and programs. Because the HOP initiative coincided with the expansion of the primary care movement that had been launched several decades earlier, the two reforming efforts had opportunities to interact. And as noted earlier, the growing awareness of the AIDS epidemic in the mid-1980s was a further powerful reminder of the limitations of therapeutic medicine.

The central question is, why did clinical disease continue to dominate the orientation of the nation's AHCs, including the 33 successful grantees of the HOP awards? True, most of the award winners made some changes in their curriculum and instituted or expanded their involvement in community partnerships, but not much else changed. As in most settings, powerful forces usually favor the status quo. In the two decades following the passage of Medicare and Medicaid, the leading research-oriented AHCs had achieved a many successes, aided by the liberal, cost-plus reimbursement policies for hospitalized patients adopted by both Medicare and private health insurance providers. Described previously were several other flows of funds that Medicare made available to the AHCs, such as the graduate medical education funds. This money was not limited to providing a low-cost professional labor supply consisting of residents and fellows. In addition, AHCs could obtain funds to compensate the teaching institutions for their higher costs that were intimately linked to their educational mission, such as the elaborate testing of patients and the concomitant slower discharge rate.

By the mid-1980s the AHCs had secured greater control over their destinies with the rapid increase in practice plan income. They speedily expanded their clinical staffs—by a factor of six compared with the pre-Medicare era. The rapidly expanding income, when combined with federal funding for biomedical research and graduate medical education, generated almost all of the additional revenue that the AHCs needed in their intensified efforts to find the causes and cures of the many diseases that they were pursuing.

But just who were the recipients of these funds? In the late 1980s a newly appointed dean of one of the nation's leading biomedical research-oriented AHCs told Eli Ginzberg about an early meeting he convened with his clinical chiefs. The dean presented some tentative ideas about changes for them to consider in the medical school's curriculum, but he quickly discovered that they had little if any interest in exploring, much less introducing, significant changes. The dean suddenly realized that the clinical chiefs, or "the barons" as he referred to them, controlled about 88 percent of the medical school's budget while he only controlled the remaining 12 percent.

In addition to money-related issues, the the prevailing professional ethos in both the United States and other developed nations further reinforced the desire to maintain the status quo. The leaders and the members of the medical profession were proud of the considerable advances that curative medicine had achieved in recent decades and greatly anticipated future gains. They had little incentive to pursue new goals when little existed in the way of precedent, methodology, or opportunity for personal accomplishment.

What other forces have encouraged the AHCs to change their priorities and methods of operation in the past decade? The brief answer is the changing health care marketplace, driven increasingly by the rapid growth of managed care. But before we explore the impact of managed care on the AHCs in the next chapter, we should note other changes in the orientation and behavior of the leading AHCs. They have begun to respond to a number of new forces, external and internal, that have been affecting their established ways in the quarter-century after the passage of Medicare, the period during which they were largely the masters of their own fate.

Notwithstanding HOP's mandate to encourage AHCs to introduce or broaden their offerings in population-based medicine, most medical students continue to be trained primarily within a patho-physiology framework during medical school. But within that essential orientation are some important modifications and changes. For example, the breakthrough advances in technology, specifically in computer software technology, introduced a considerable shift in how students learn. Large classroom lectures are declining and being replaced by more emphasis on self-learning and small group discussions.

The managed care changes in the health care marketplace have led most research-oriented AHCs to provide residencies in family medicine. More graduates are selecting a primary care specialty when they begin their residency training—no wonder that an increasing number of students have chosen this path in the past four years. Because medical students are willing to commit many years to preparing for practice and are willing to assume heavy debt during their training, they are clearly sensitive to the ways in which practice opportunities are changing. Even the most inward looking, research-oriented AHCs must be at least selectively responsive to the changing attitudes and behavior of their undergraduate students and residents.

When we shift focus from the areas of specialization to the numbers and types of physicians who should be admitted and trained, the AHCs have not been at the forefront of advocating major reforms. With their students and residents remaining a source of cheap labor and additional revenue, the AHCs mostly have favored the status quo and have not campaigned for broad-based cutbacks in enrollments. However, as previously noted, selected leadership groups, including the AAMC, the AMA, and COGME, have recently begun to press Congress to cut back on the number of international graduates admitted to the United States for Medicare-paid residency training.

Most AHCs have been equally slow to respond to other challenges, largely because aggressive action would have led to serious difficulties in staffing and expenditures. Since World War II, for example, medical students and residents have received most of their clinical training in the major teaching hospital of the AHC and its affiliated teaching hospitals. Although patient treatment has shifted considerably to ambulatory care sites since 1980, until recently most AHCs have not moved more of their training to ambulatory sites. Issues of curriculum, patient exposure, and simple traditionalism, as well as costs have all played a part in the centers' plodding pace.

The traditionalism of most AHCs, especially those among the leaders in biomedical research, is also evident in their slowness in refocusing attention to the oldest patient group. This remains true despite the growing emphasis in the leading medical journals on the striking numbers of people who are surviving into their eighties, nineties, and even past their one-hundredth birthday. Nor have the increasing efforts of the Robert Wood Johnson Foundation to shift the teaching emphasis from acute to chronic care had much effect. Admittedly, health-illness patterns of the oldest subgroups of the population represent a paradox of sorts; many within this group are more focused on keeping active than on seeking medical attention, and many of those who do seek medical attention patronize so-called alternative practitioners.

But if the healthy oldest group presents relatively few challenges to modern medicine, the same is not true for the steadily growing numbers between age 55 and 85 who are afflicted with one or more chronic conditions and need ongoing interaction with the medical care system. Although most AHCs have begun to pay more attention to geriatrics, relatively few medical schools and residency programs have made more than minor curriculum adjustments to shift their preoccupation from acute to chronic diseases. As medical schools and residency programs become more attentive and responsive to the growing importance of chronic diseases, the classic pattern for delivering medical care involving one patient interacting with one physician will require modification. AHCs face a major challenge of restructuring the delivery of medical care services to make use of an organized team approach. Under this structure the physician would head a team comprising midlevel medical and other personnel consisting of nurses, technicians, physical therapists, social workers, and others. The team would collectively provide the complex range of preventive, therapeutic, and rehabilitative services that many chronic patients require from the time that they are first diagnosed for conditions requiring ongoing medical attention.

AHCs face one more high-priority challenge that most of them have yet to recognize or have made only initial efforts to confront and resolve. This issue returns to a central concern of the HOP initiative that sought to shift the focus of medical care in the direction of prevention and away from an almost total preoccupation with acute care intervention. An ever-increasing proportion of the population is living past the Medicare eligibility age. Average elderly American males are now living into their late seventies and American women into their early eighties. The citizenry needs to be encouraged early on — and reminded frequently — that their good health depends less on physician intervention than on the lifestyles that they pursue throughout their lives. Although neither physicians nor patients will aggressively pursue such a shift in focus from physician interaction to self-responsibility, such a refocusing is long overdue.

The explosive growth of managed care could conceivably speed such a refocusing. But no matter what happens during the next stages in the managed care revolution, the AHCs will be forced to react. It is possible, if not likely, that we could see a speedy shift in emphasis from acute to chronic care, a change that will be reflected in significant revisions in the training of medical students and residents and the future practice of physicians.

5
The Impacts of Managed Care

In this chapter we assess the impacts of managed care and Medicaid managed care on the AHCs and the urban poor. The outlook for the evolution of managed care remains uncertain, hence we begin by telling the story of the managed care revolution since the early 1980s, when the enrollment shift from fee-for-service insurance to managed care started to accelerate. We continue by looking at developments in the 1990s, when the shift to managed care intensified and state Medicaid managed care enrollments also accelerated. But first we offer a brief summary of events that contributed to the managed care revolution that has increasingly dominated the past two decades.

The beginnings of prepaid group practice arrangements can be traced to 1929 in Los Angeles, and its post–World War II expansion is closely linked to the growth of Kaiser Permanente. Kaiser Permanente started as a nonprofit organization characterized by ownership of its hospitals, group practice sites, and arrangements that negotiated exclusive contracts with most of its physician staffs. Our focus, however, is primarily the policy developments during the 1970s. In 1973, Congress passed the Health Maintenance Organization Act, which offered federal subsidies for the establishment and expansion of nonprofit HMOs. The newly created organizations had relatively few takers for various reasons, including the excessive number of conditions that applicants had to meet. In a separate but related action the following year, Congress passed the Employee Retirement Insurance Security Act (ERISA), which reinforced the barriers that had prevented the states from regulating private insurance companies that dealt with employers operating in multiple states. Although the new statute was primarily intended to improve federal oversight over corporate employee pension benefits, it also created opportunities for large and midsized companies to self-insure and provide health care benefits for their employees. A few of the companies that did self-insure early on paid more attention to the rapid increases in their health care benefit costs. These increases had become more dramatic with the high rate of inflation affecting the economy at large and, in particular, its health care sector.

But more than inflation, the major contributor-to the explosive growth of managed care was the consequence of the rapid increases in health care services for the American people after the passage of Medicare and Medicaid. For a time, no one paid close attention to the rapidly increasing costs and how to moderate them. The bills that were incurred for the delivery of expanded medical services were sent either to employers or to the federal and state governments, all of which paid on demand with little or no review. With the lowering or removal of the preexisting controls on health care outlays, some new form of overseeing future costs was urgently needed and inevitable. Admittedly, because the newly entitled Medicare population, AHCs and community hospitals, physicians, and other health care personnel prospered during this time, the reinstitution of dollar controls was expectedly at first ignored and later delayed. But some form of "managed care" was inevitable by the beginning of the 1980s.

Admissions to acute care hospitals began to drop radically as a result of the severe recession of 1980–81. This reduction was intensified by medical technology advances that enabled physicians to treat more patients in an ambulatory setting. Not surprisingly, southern California, where these conditions had become most pronounced, took the lead in expanding the numbers of patients in managed care. The growing excess of hospital capacity in the region provided one spur. The increasing free appointment time in the schedules of some specialists was another. The earlier, greater exposure of California residents to prepaid systems of care was yet another. And the willingness of the medical profession to experiment with the newly emerging independent physician association (IPA)/network system of managed care was a further precipitant. This last development meant that private practitioners could add managed care patients to their roster and bill the managed care plan below their established charges while continuing to treat and charge their private patients as they had previously. Savings were not limited to shaving the fee paid to the IPA physician for taking care of the plan's patients. In addition, the managed care plan was often able to obtain significant discounts from underutilized hospitals by contracting to send them additional patients.

The IPA/network was an attractive method of bringing sizable numbers of fee-for-service patients into a managed care arrangement. The IPA model, in contrast to the staff-group model such as Kaiser-Permanente, did not require large capital outlays for the purchase or building of a hospital facility, nor did it require physicians to join and practice as salaried members of a large group practice. The IPA approach could be grafted onto the existing model of private practice.

Although the conditions in southern California were increasingly ripe at this time for the growth of managed care arrangements, this was not the case elsewhere in the country. Most other regions had had little or no prior exposure to prepaid medical care, and the capacity of the acute care hospital system outside of California was not yet in serious surplus. In fact, occasionally the reverse was true, as was the case in New York City in the the late 1980s.

Moreover, businesses had varying degrees of interest and concern with rising health care costs. Employers in the Twin Cities were among the first seeking to rationalize the health care sector. In contrast, along the Atlantic coast—home to many of the nation's leading AHCs—the business community paid relatively little attention to the steady rise in their premiums until the late 1980s or early 1990s.

To expand and maintain profitability, managed care plans needed to attract and retain employees. The increase in managed care plans' membership depended, in turn, on employers encouraging or mandating their employees to shift from fee-for-service to managed care plan coverage. Such a shift could save 15 percent or so in the cost of coverage. Because of these savings, most managed care plans were able to reduce the rate of increase in the premiums that employers had been paying when their employees were enrolled in fee-for-service coverage.

With the stock market booming (except during the 1987 selloff) and with prospective continued good earnings, the more aggressive managed care companies could obtain additional capital relatively easily through borrowing and issuing stock to speed their growth. By 1994, 90 percent of the for-profit managed care plans listed on the New York Stock Exchange reported profits for the year. But the reports for the following two years—while the stock market continued its upward climb—were less favorable. The reason is simple: the number of the below-65 population that could be shifted from fee-for-service coverage to managed care plans had dwindled.

As increasing numbers of the population joined managed care plans throughout the 1980s—and more particularly during the early 1990s—the leading research-oriented AHCs began to feel the effects in both revenues and overall operations, and these shifts greatly affected their relations to the urban poor. In previous chapters we discussed how the financial position of most research-oriented AHCs improved notably after the passage of Medicare and Medicaid, and they could pursue their high-priority goals. For the leading centers this meant that they could focus more on biomedical research and providing increasingly sophisticated high-tech treatment to seriously ill patients. Further, the clinical staffs of the leading AHCs expanded their practice plan activities through treating increasing numbers of paying patients. The urban poor rarely command the attention of their nearby AHC. True, many of the urban poor continued to seek treatment from the emergency rooms of their neighboring AHCs, which, by federal law (COBRA), had to assess and, if necessary, stabilize patients before referring them to alternate providers. With few exceptions, the nongovernment-owned AHCs sought to limit the number of the urban poor—particularly the uninsured—whom they admitted for in-patient care.

As the numbers and percentages of the previously enrolled population in fee-for-service coverage were increasingly shifted over to a managed care arrangement, this shift became a more serious challenge for the financial well-being of the AHCs. Because a principal goal of managed care plans is to reduce unnecessarily high-cost services to their members, most managed care plans reduced referrals for inpatient care. Advances in technology enabled an increasing number of procedures—including complex procedures—to be performed in an ambulatory setting.

This was only the first adverse effect of managed care on the revenues of the AHCs. Particularly hard hit were the leading research AHCs that had a pricing structure of about 30 percent above other well-staffed and well-functioning community hospitals. In many locations managed care plans were able to negotiate reductions in surcharges from their local AHC. In addition, some managed care plans were able to exert pressure on the AHCs to reduce patients' length of stay. And many managed care plans refused to authorize payment for costly procedures that they categorized as "experimental."

Various preexisting conditions influenced the extent to which leading AHCs came under increasing financial pressure as a result of the large-scale expansion of managed care enrollments, especially in the 1990s. One example was the level of domination of managed care arrangements in the the local market area. Another key condition was the ability of the AHC leadership to exploit alternative revenue possibilities to enable the centers to continue their complex activities, including those that required cross-subsidization.

Not unexpectedly, most AHCs paid insufficient attention to inefficiencies that developed while they were operating under a favorable revenue environment. Faced with increasingly aggressive behavior on the part of large payers, especially the rapidly growing managed care plans, more hospital CEOs focused renewed attention and energy on reengineering and cost reductions. In just a few years some cut millions of dollars in expenditures out of their previously swollen budgets. Others reexamined their special strengths and sought to build on them by expanding services that might attract additional paying patients who needed the specialized services that an AHC could provide.

Other heads of AHC hospitals, recognizing the continuing, strong shifts from inpatient to ambulatory care treatment settings, decided that they had much to gain by getting in front of this trend rather than lagging behind it. Several leading AHCs between Boston and Baltimore, as well as centers in other regions, sought either to develop alliances with existing physician groups practicing in affluent suburbs or to seed their own groups there. The centers anticipated that such a move would ensure an expanded number of referrals for hospital consultation and for inpatient treatment at their respective institutions. Another step was to form a network relationship with selected urban and suburban hospitals, because many teaching and community hospitals are located within reasonable distances from AHCs. A growing number of CEOs of leading medical centers have been actively engaged in securing these arrangements with outlying hospitals. The facilities gain prestige from their association with a leading medical center. Their residency programs are strengthened, and their clinical staffs receive increased exposure and support. For their part, the AHCs expect these outliers to refer a considerable number of patients for consultation, assessment, and inpatient treatment—all of which add to the AHCs' revenue base. But the main strength of such arrangements is the increasing parity concerning contract negotiations with insurers. Few of these networking arrangements have moved beyond the early stages of arm's-length association to major integrations between AHCs and their outlying affiliates. Most successful suburban hospitals have been reluctant to sacrifice their independence and integrate their boards, management structures, clinical staffs, and capital assets with the much larger AHC. Some outright consolidations and mergers have occurred, resulting in a fully integrated network, but the networking arrangements mostly stop far short of full integration.

Before we shift the focus to Medicaid managed care we need to briefly consider the changes that Congress introduced in passing the Balanced Budget Act of 1997, because they affect the future structure and operation of Medicare + Choice, the alternative to the traditional fee-for-service Medicare arrangement. Clearly much awaits the development of the detailed regulations that will accompany and eventually reshape the much altered Medicare system. But even at this early date we can recognize some potential impacts of the new structure on the future well-being of the AHC.

As noted earlier, the much-improved financial position of the AHCs dates from the start of the Medicare program in July 1966. In the early 1970s the Medicare-eligible population was increased with the extension of coverage to patients of any age suffering from end-stage renal disease. The lists were further augmented with the enrollment of the permanently disabled two years following their injury. And in 1989, while canceling most of the provisions of the Medicare catastrophic legislation of the preceding year, Congress retained the provision to assist some elderly beyond the very poor whom Medicaid was already covering. Under this amendment, this population was jointly covered by Medicaid and Medicare, with Medicaid covering their deductibles, copayments, and out-patient drugs.

Two additional changes dating from the early 1980s also affected AHCs. First, Congress agreed that HMOs could enroll Medicare patients for whom the federal government's reimbursement rate was set at 95 percent of the average of that geographic area's Medicare fee-for-service expenditures. Later studies revealed that, because of self-selection, the costs of treating the healthier Medicare cohorts in HMOs increased the federal government's outlay 5 percent above what it would have paid had this group remained within fee-for-service arrangements. But the demonstration had a significant payoff. Even before the expanded scope of managed care arrangements came to dominate U.S. health care in the 1990s, individuals in good health could profit by selecting or remaining in an HMO once they became Medicare eligible and thereby gaining access to a range of supplementary benefits that Medicare did not provide its fee-for-service beneficiaries. By the end of 1999 about 7 million Medicare enrollees belonged to a managed care plan, an approximately 125 percent increase from 1993.

In introducing Medicare + Choice, the Balanced Budget Act, while leaving the long-established fee-for-service system in place, offered Medicare beneficiaries many alternatives. They could enroll in an HMO with or without options for going out of the network. Other choices included preferred provider organizations (PPOs), provider-sponsored organizations (PSOs), and medical savings accounts (MSAs) as a limited demonstration. Vicki Gottlieb, an analyst from the National Senior Citizens Law Center, has speculated that "the changes began the transformation of Medicare from a defined benefit program . . . to a defined contribution program." Her interpretation and forecast may prove to be correct given the continuing pressure on Congress to moderate the out-year costs of the Medicare program.

We also need to include in our discussion the recently expanded coverage that Medicare has undertaken to pay for home health care benefits. According to the General Accounting Office, the costs for this program have increased from an estimated $2.9 billion in 1990 to $21.9 billion in fiscal 1998.

How are the above changes, especially Medicare + Choice, likely to affect the revenue position of the AHC in the near-middle term? A conservative estimate suggests that these innovations point to a decline in the proportion of Medicare revenues to total AHC revenues. Determining the extent of this decline will primarily be the rate at which Medicare eligibles join and remain in an HMO. We should remember the important role that practice plan income plays in AHC revenues—about 50 percent in the leading research-oriented centers. The potential future rapid enrollment of Medicare patients in HMOs carries with it the threat of reduced referrals of their members for both ambulatory and inpatient care to AHCs. Accompanying reduced referrals is added pressure on the future revenue position of the AHCs. Furthermore, the average per capita costs were calculated regionwide to include the teaching (graduate medical education) costs of AHCs, but until recently those dollars were not obligated to go proportionately back to the AHC.

Although the open questions affecting the future of Medicare are only beginning to be recognized and confronted, an increasing number of states are moving aggressively to enroll many or most of their Medicaid eligibles into a managed care arrangement. In 1981, when Arizona finally joined the federal-state Medicaid system—the last state to do so—the federal government granted it a waiver to enroll selected Medicaid eligibles in a managed care system. However, not until the early to mid-1990s did an increasing number of states seek and obtain waivers from the federal government to experiment with moving some or many of their Medicaid-eligible individuals into one or another type of managed care plan. A few states believed that such action would enable them to save money that could be used to enroll some or most of the uninsured while at the same time meeting their ongoing obligations to their Medicaid-eligible population.

Although we focus our attention on Medicaid managed care largely on the post-1990 initiatives led by Oregon, Tennessee, New York, and other states, we should remember that one of the most ambitious state initiatives goes back to the early 1970s. During Ronald Reagan's first term as governor of California, the state launched a major effort to enroll large numbers of Medi-Cal enrollees into managed care. Many sponsors of the new managed care plans, however, were upstart entrepreneurs looking to make a quick dollar, and the plans lacked the necessary infrastructure supports, including adequate numbers of physicians willing to treat the newly enrolled. The effort folded shortly after being launched. A decade later a similar effort was made in Chicago's inner city to enroll substantial numbers of Medicaid eligibles when several new managed care plans sought to establish or strengthen themselves in that area. But the outcome, though not as bleak as the earlier effort in California, left much to be desired.

In the early 1980s, New York City mayor Ed Koch, with the support of Governor Hugh Carey, sought to launch a modest prepaid Medicaid enrollment effort. Koch attempted to shift into the plan some members of the Puerto Rican community in East Harlem who had long been cared for in a public hospital (Metropolitan

Hospital) that was threatened with closure. The plan provoked the ire of large numbers of the Medicaid eligibles who didn't want to lose their existing freedom of choice to select their physicians. The opposition, which included local political leaders, caused both Koch and Carey to back off. Koch ultimately found a way to ensure the continued operation of Metropolitan Hospital.

During the second half of the 1980s, Philadelphia launched a sizable Medicaid managed care plan with help from the state. This plan, recruiting the participation of several of the inner city AHCs, achieved a membership of some 100,000 by 1989 and impressed experts with the quality of care that it delivered. The state provided liberal financing, which was augmented by a primary care grant from the Robert Wood Johnson Foundation. The Philadelphia effort provided good care to many Medicaid enrollees. It also served many of the uninsured poor who lived in the same or nearby low-income neighborhoods. However, in the late 1990s the state legislature significantly reduced funding for the city, and the plan faced great difficulties in continuing to care for the same number of uninsured patients.

Although the federal government had paved the way for the enrollment of Medicaid eligibles into managed care plans in 1981, this option did not become a priority for most states until the 1990s. For one thing, conditions were strict. HCFA carefully reviewed all state requests for waivers to ensure that the existing rights of the Medicaid population were protected, especially if a state planned the enforced enrollment of Medicaid recipients into managed care. For another, state officials were aware of the HMOs' reluctance to enroll Medicaid populations. The early group health maintenance organizations, such as Kaiser-Permanente and the Health Insurance Plan of New York, assumed that Medicaid eligibles were high-cost patients and avoided enrolling more than small numbers of them. Moreover, the HMOs anticipated that these patients would be difficult to serve because of the disinclination of most physicians to practice in areas where the poor were concentrated. Not until the late 1980s and early 1990s did private sector managed care enrollments reach a level to substantiate that such arrangements were no longer the exception but increasingly the norm.

A third factor was the passage of a series of new federal Medicaid mandates in the late 1980s requiring the states to raise additional matching funds. This action forced governors and state legislative leaders to focus increasing attention on ways to contain their Medicaid costs that were increasing steeply in the face of rapid health care inflation. With few if any alternatives facing them, most states not surprisingly have opted for Medicaid managed care. What's more, states have not been forced to seek waivers since 1997.

Don Boyd of the Rockefeller Institute of Government in Albany, New York, has investigated variations among the states in the percentage of their spending for the Medicaid-covered poor and Medicaid enrollees, both overall and as a percentage of their poverty population, with state spending and enrollments indexed to the U.S. average. According to his analysis, with respect to state spending per poor person, Rhode Island, Massachusetts, and New York are the leaders, spending about twice as much as the U.S. average. New Mexico, Alabama, Oklahoma, and Texas spend the least, between .55 and .58 of the national average. In the category of spending per Medicaid enrollee, the District of Columbia and New York are just below 2.0. They are followed by Massachusetts and Rhode Island in the 1.7 and high 1.6 ranges, respectively. On ranking Medicaid enrollees as a percentage of the poor population, Vermont leads with 1.80 and Tennessee is second with a ranking of 1.66. As one might expect, the lowest spending states per poor person are among the lowest spending states per Medicaid enrollee.

Boyd offers a number of broad conclusions about the variations in his data sets. He demonstrates that the northeast states spend considerably more per poor person and per Medicaid enrollee than do most southern and western states. His analysis shows that the differentials in spending are foreshadowed in considerable part by the per capita income of the different states. Further, he points out how differential cost structures in the provision of high-cost hospital and nursing home care are also important factors. But possibly the most important conclusion to be drawn from these data is that wide differences exist in both the extent and depth of coverage, even though the federal-state program has been operating for over 30 years, with the federal government providing between 50 and 83 percent of funding.

Oregon made a serious commitment in the early 1990s to enroll all of its Medicaid-eligible population in managed care, hoping to cover increasing numbers of the uninsured with some rationalization of service delivery and associated economies. The state has made some progress, but not as much or as fast as it had initially anticipated.

Tennessee, facing major budgetary challenges in the early 1990s, also moved energetically to shift all of its Medicaid eligibles into managed care. It also restructured its dollar flow to include a large number of its low-income, uninsured poor in its new coverage plan. The state encountered substantial opposition from physicians as well as from teaching hospitals and other health care providers that were adversely affected, but it has stayed the course, making only modest changes and corrections. Despite the lack of an in-depth assessment of Tennessee's ambitious effort, this program has been the target of increasing criticism.

As of the end of 1999, none of the larger industrialized states such as California, Illinois, or New York had made substantial progress in moving a significant proportion of their Medicaid-eligible population into a managed care model. The planned timetable for the transfer in California had earlier been put on hold. In Illinois disagreements continue between the legislative leaders in Springfield and the political leadership in Chicago, with little action to date. New York State, having committed itself in 1991 to transfer at least half of all Medicaid eligibles by the mid-1990s into a managed care plan, fell far short of its goal. After prolonged negotiations with HCFA, the state sought a new waiver, which it obtained in 1997 after a long delay. This agreement set a very ambitious goal for 1999, aimed at enrolling most Medicaid eligibles into managed care by 2000. But New York State's ambitious schedule may not be met. For one, total New York City enrollment in Medicaid managed care, a figure that grew from 100,000 in 1993 to 500,000 by mid-1995, declined to 395,000 as of early 1999. Several factors contributed to this decline. The city lacked a sufficient number of physicians to care for the enrolled population. In the face of the legislature's reduction in Medicaid contract payments, several for-profit managed care companies have withdrawn from the New York City market. For another, the considerable adverse publicity that followed upon the enrollment scandals of 1995 brought the earlier enrollment effort to a sudden halt.

Further problems complicate the overall situation. About 70 percent of the total Medicaid population consists of mothers and children. Most are single mothers, and many have been on welfare for considerable periods of time. This population generally is healthy and relatively easy to enroll and treat so long as they can contact and communicate with practitioners. But this is not always the case. Although a few of the more aggressive managed care providers have mounted special efforts to provide accessible treatment sites, many physicians and other health care personnel have sought to avoid treating Medicaid eligibles. In addition, repeated reports of misunderstandings have occurred because Medicaid enrollees did not secure prior approval from their managed care plan to use the local hospital's emergency room after hours or over the weekend when their primary care practitioner was unavailable. Because these patients had used the facilities of their local hospital in the past, they continued to do so, particularly if and when their managed care plan failed to be responsive. These and other administrative and financing challenges need to be addressed and resolved. But the treatment needs of Medicaid-eligible mothers and children enrolled in managed care plans do not present particular hurdles once families are linked to accessible physicians. Although not an easy task, it is possible.

The more serious challenge, to which no large state has yet been able to provide a definitive response, is the extent to which the newly expanded Medicaid managed care plans will be able to care effectively and economically for the most vulnerable Medicaid patients. This population includes the disabled, the elderly, the blind, and the chronically ill. Although they total only about one third of all Medicaid eligibles, these patients account for almost 70 percent of all Medicaid outlays. Dr. Sara Rosenbaum and her colleagues at the George Washington Medical Center in Washington, D.C., have investigated new arrangements between states are contractors that are willing to assume responsibility on a fixed-cost basis for providing most if not all the services that the seriously impaired Medicaid-eligible population requires. In the past, the range of services that this population needed usually involved the participation of a number of state, and sometimes local, government agencies, and most or all of the services were paid on a fee-for-service basis. Under the new approach, the state enters into a single contract with a managed care plan that assumes responsibility for providing the gamut, sometimes with carve outs (subcontracting certain services to specialized providers) of all services that the enrolled population requires. If contractors perform as promised, the states and their officials will be better off because they will no longer be directly responsible for providing the multiple services needed by this difficult population. But as emphasized in the early assessments of the new contracting approaches, nothing is easy when it comes to collecting and evaluating the evidence to judge the accomplishment of these Medicaid managed care plans.

It is difficult to tell if these plans are fulfilling their written commitments to serve any or all of these patient groups. Equally if not more important is whether these vulnerable populations are receiving the same or higher level of care as they received earlier through various fee-for-service arrangements. As of 1999, the jury is still out, and it is likely to remain out for quite a while, given that only a few of the smaller states—Hawaii, Arizona, Oregon, and Tennessee—have a track record that can be assessed. None of the larger states is very far along in transferring their disabled Medicaid populations into managed care arrangements. With strong pressures on state legislators to control their Medicaid expenditures, and with private contractors responsible for the delivery of a galaxy of complex services, the room for slippage is considerable.

Judging from the revenue positions of the key teaching hospitals, most of the leading AHCs have thus far been able to absorb the impacts of managed care with just a few exceptions, such as San Diego and the Twin Cities. AHCs have been able to continue to obtain substantial surcharges for their inpatient admissions (or to find some alternative source of additional revenue) to help them continue to cross-subsidize their education, research, and charity functions. But since Medicare + Choice and Medicaid managed care for the elderly and the disabled are still largely on the drawing board, their impact on the revenue position of the AHCs won't be known for several more years. Furthermore, the state-by-state variability is impressive both in terms of the percentage of managed care penetration and the rates for capitation.

Clues from both the more- and less-vulnerable AHCs, however, can help provide an early view of how the urban AHCs see their changing relations to the urban poor. After Medicare and Medicaid greatly improved their financial position, most AHCs no longer needed the urban poor to support their leading programs. The relationship they maintained resulted from the continuing heavy use of their emergency room by their low-income neighbors. In addition, the Medicaid population was admitted for inpatient care at a moderate rate.

Once inpatient admissions to acute care hospitals started their steep decline in the early 1980s, some AHCs adopted a more hospitable view about accepting Medicaid patients for inpatient care. In most instances these patients filled beds that otherwise would have remained vacant. At New York City's Presbyterian Hospital, an AHC located in a low-income area, Medicaid had become the single largest payer by 1997, accounting for over 40 percent of the hospital's revenue.

Even before the passage of the Balanced Budget Act of 1997 and the accelerated effort of many states to implement Medicaid managed care, a number of AHCs began to explore how they could develop closer relations with their neighborhood poor. This was especially true along the East coast. These facilities recognized that both they and the local poor might profit from such efforts. As early as the mid-1980s, Presbyterian Hospital took initial steps to seed primary care practices and clinics in surrounding areas. It offered selected local physicians the opportunity to admit to the hospital. More recently the AHC began experimenting with advance practice nurses who have admission privileges to Presbyterian's Allen Pavillion, a fully owned community hospital in northern Manhattan. In association with two other hospitals in this area, one voluntary and the other public, Presbyterian is developing a conjointly owned HMO aimed at increasing its ability to care for more Medicaid eligibles. Among other potential benefits, Presbyterian anticipates that, if the HMO grows, the AHC will profit from a larger number of admissions for inpatient care.

Johns Hopkins, situated in the midst of a large low-income population, has long sought an appropriate balance between services to its poor neighbors while continuing to attract large numbers of the well-insured from surrounding areas as well as from more distant locations. For the third time in the past 10 years it is starting an HMO, concluding that it cannot afford to turn its back on the potential revenue that an HMO with heavy Medicaid enrollment could contribute to the hospital's budget. In this case the amount is estimated to be 12 to 15 percent of hospital revenues.

Certainly revenue flows have been, and will continue to be, critical in enabling AHCs to fulfill their multiple missions. But the question of the relationship between the urban AHCs and the urban poor has other dimensions as well. One example stems from the changing needs of the medical schools to expand their opportunities for training more students and residents in ambulatory settings. The recent trends of fewer admissions to teaching hospitals, and the accelerated discharge of patients admitted for inpatient care, raise serious questions about the future training sites for medical students and residents.

For some time, conventional wisdom among medical educators has been that medical students and residents need much more of their training to be conducted in ambulatory care sites. To date, however, most urban-based AHCs have had difficulty in expanding such training opportunities because of a shortage of suitable sites and the associated higher costs. In a few locations, however, such as Boston, the AHCs have established ties with community ambulatory sites. Another problem has been finding physicians ready to practice among the poor, but one possible solution provides an opportunity for both the AHCs and the poor. By forging relationships with the urban poor, AHCs can address their need for more ambulatory sites for the training of physicians and other health care workers while responding to the need of managed care plans by making personnel available to provide care for the poor.

Two other patient groups increase the potential for closer bonding between the AHCs and the urban poor. First, the Robert Wood Johnson Foundation has insisted that a major challenge to the U.S. health care system is to direct greater attention to patients with chronic illness, a high proportion of whom continue to live in their own homes or apartments. If true, the AHCs face a serious challenge of providing opportunities not only for their physicians in training but also for other members of the health care team, especially nurses, therapists, technicians, and social workers, to explore new approaches for taking care of the chronically ill. AHCs that recognize and respond to this challenge and opportunity will seek to establish and strengthen their ties to their low-income neighbors. The second group is the uninsured, most of whom are poor. As a consequence of the growing pressures on reducing the surcharges that the AHCs were long able to command, approximately 30 percent for inpatient care, cross-subsidization of the care of the uninsured and other urban poor is definitely threatened. Many leading AHCs will be fortunate if they can continue to obtain a 10–15 percent surcharge. Such reductions suggest that, without innovation, the centers will have less opportunity to care for the uninsured. In New York City the uninsured number is approximately 1.5 million out of a population of some 7.5 million. And because the passage of welfare legislation in 1996 makes public assistance a time-limited government benefit, the number of uninsured will likely increase.

Another financial concern is the lower payments made to certain urban hospitals that are located in low-income neighborhoods and that treat disproportionate numbers of the poor. The federal government has made sizable additional sums available—nearly $18 billion in previous years—as annual "disproportionate share payments" for compensating reimbursement to these hospitals. With the passage of the Balanced Budget Act of 1997 Congress reduced the federal allocation. A more serious threat to the future provision of essential medical care for the uninsured is the vulnerability of "essential community providers" (ECPs). These agencies primarily are community clinics that had previously cared for large numbers of Medicaid enrollees and that stretched their Medicaid payments to enable them to provide care for many of the local uninsured. With most states now stepping up efforts to forcibly enroll many or most of their Medicaid population in managed care plans, many ECPs are under threat. They may find that a significant proportion of their former Medicaid clientele has been redirected into a managed care plan that has not entered into a contract with them, denying them a significant part of their former income flow. This, in turn, makes it much more difficult for them to provide care for the uninsured or, in some cases, even to remain in operation. And for the reasons that we have reviewed earlier, inner-city AHCs will find it very difficult—if not impossible—to pick up the slack because they likewise are facing a more straitened financial outlook.

A final point to consider in the triangle of managed care, the AHCs, and the urban poor concerns early exposure of physicians to a managed care environment. Many analysts have observed how it would be useful for medical school undergraduates and graduates to experience the operations of managed care plans. After all, they most likely will be practicing in a managed care environment, albeit probably a changing one, during much, most, or all of their careers. To the extent that the medical leadership agree on the usefulness of such early exposure to managed care, the urban AHC should consider, sooner rather than later, how it might provide such an environment for its students and residents. Entering into the ownership of, or a partnership with, an HMO or other managed care organization could make good sense. Such an arrangement might make it easier for the AHC to meet future financial and professional challenges while it expands its health care services to the urban poor.

6
The Next Decade—2000–2010

In this concluding chapter we assess likely developments for the next ten years. The year 2010 marks an important point in the evolution of our nation's health care delivery system because it coincides with Medicare eligibility of the first of the post–World War II baby-boom generation (unless Congress acts first to alter the age of eligibility). But first we will examine the transformations that occurred during the last decade of the twentieth century in restructuring the functioning of prestigious AHCs, the changing conditions affecting different groups of the urban poor as they continued to seek access to ambulatory and inpatient hospital care, and the interactions between the most sophisticated and most vulnerable groups in the health care arena. This analysis assumes that the federal government, the dominant participant in altering the boundaries of our evolving health care system, is unlikely to take the initiative to introduce national health insurance, an effort that failed most recently in 1994. Nevertheless, the prospect of yet another national effort to pass universal health insurance coverage during the coming decade must be considered in assessing the possible structure of our evolving health care sector.

More than any other development affecting both the AHCs and the urban poor during the 1990s was the failure of the Clinton health reform proposals in 1994. Many believed that the competitive market would ultimately moderate the rise in health care costs; reduce excess hospital capacity; bring the future supply of physicians both in numbers and types into better alignment with patient requirements; and, above all, expand the enrollments of the population in managed care arrangements, which promised to provide a better quality of care at lower costs.

In the last five years of the twentieth century even the nation's most prestigious AHCs were under increasing revenue pressures as the flow of patients requiring inpatient care continued to decline, managed care companies negotiated lower charges, and the federal government passed the Balanced Budget Act of 1997, which reduces prospective reimbursements for Medicare recipients by $115 billion over a five-year period. The one bright spot for the leading research-oriented AHCs was the bipartisan support in Washington to increase federal funding for biomedical research by 50 percent over the next five years. Policy decisions on several other important fronts remained on hold, particularly concerning physicians and other health personnel in whose education and clinical training the AHCs play a leading role. We should also mention selective organizational realignments, especially on the east and west Coasts, of AHCs in the same market area such as Boston, New York, and San Francisco, to help strengthen their future economic position.

These recent changes notwithstanding, the leading AHCs were characterized throughout the 1990s by their marked continuity in organization and performance despite changing health policy and market conditions. They continued to focus most of their organizational strengths, financial resources, and intellectual capital on pursuing their priority goals: specialist training, biomedical research aimed at finding improved treatment and cures for a range of diseases, and capital outlays aimed at improving patient care.

In shifting attention to our other primary focus group—the urban poor—the following are some highlights of the past decade. Despite the strong national economy and, in particular, the decline in unemployment, many of the urban poor continued to encounter difficulties in obtaining access to the health care system. During this time the number of uninsured increased to more than 43 million, a new high. That figure is likely to grow even higher once the time limits for federal-state support for persons on welfare, legislated in 1996, become fully operative.

The 1990s have also seen most states move aggressively to enroll most of their Medicaid-eligible persons into managed care plans to save money and provide better care. Some of the less-populous states, such as Hawaii, Arizona, Oregon, and Tennessee, have developed a reasonable track record, but the more heavily populated states, such as California, New York, and Illinois, have encountered difficulties in transferring the chronically ill, the disabled, and the blind from fee-for-service coverage into managed care. But a growing number of both small and large states were reasonably far advanced by 1999 in enrolling low-income Medicaid mothers and their children into managed care plans.

To complete this retrospective, we will offer a few comments on the changing relations between the AHCs and the urban poor during the 1990s. Interactions between the two generally were limited at the outset of the decade and were not markedly different 10 years later. Because of the overall decline in the use of their inpatient facilities, most large teaching hospitals, particularly those located in low-income urban areas, came to welcome Medicaid admissions. And a number of essential community providers (ECP) either joined existing managed care plans or started their own to protect their Medicaid revenue stream that they have long used to care not only for Medicaid eligibles but also many of the uninsured. A summary description of the late 1990s would include the spectacular growth of enrollments in managed care plans; rising customer discontent with managed care; no major policy changes at the leading AHCs; and growing difficulty of the urban poor in securing the medical care they need, when they need it, and, especially, from physicians who have treated them previously. Neither the AHC nor the urban poor was more than marginally affected by events in the 1990s.

The next ten years may hold much more in the way of change for both groups. To begin, the leading research-oriented AHCs would certainly feel the effects if Congress approves legislation to increase federal funding for biomedical research by 50 percent from the current level of $18 billion within the next five years. Such an action would strengthen and reinforce the key values that have dominated the leading AHCs surely since the implementation of Medicare. Moreover, a growing number of the research-oriented AHCs have entered into new arrangements and alliances with selected for-profit pharmaceutical and medical supply companies, a trend that will probably intensify. If these new collaborative arrangements prove successful, as is likely, the long-in-place high-tech efforts of the leading AHCs will be strengthened.

As more Americans live longer, and as the nation's income and wealth distribution likely continues to be characterized by a significant minority able to obtain the most sophisticated and costly medical, surgical, and rehabilitative treatments, the leading AHCs can anticipate that their high-tech treatment modalities will continue to be in demand. Here is further reinforcement of the dominant AHC ethos, with both its research and its patient care missions likely to be revalidated.

The forecast for the third part of the AHC tripod, the future educational mission, is less clear. The number of U.S. allopathic medical schools (124), as well as enrollments, has not changed over most of the past two decades, with the conspicuous exception of the closure of Oral Roberts in 1990–91. Despite occasional proposals to decrease the number of admissions to U.S. medical schools, as well as the number of medical schools in operation by approximately 20 percent, little evidence points to early action. State legislatures, which sponsor about 60 percent of all U.S. medical schools, would be hard-pressed to reduce enrollments, much less close one or more medical schools, confronted as they are within their jurisdictions by areas that lack an adequate supply of physicians. And as the Allegheny breakup helped to remind us, one of the first challenges that was successfully met was to find a new home for the Allegheny Medical College in Philadelphia, also home to 6 medical schools, including the nation's largest osteopathic school. Without data that point to significant under- or unemployment of actively practicing physicians, or major employment obstacles for recent residents, our pluralistic health care system, which continues to look askance at extensions of government powers, likely will not act soon to reduce the output of physicians.

But if changes in the supply of physicians graduating from U.S. medical schools remain problematic in the decade ahead, the same may not hold true for the generalist-specialist issue. Ever stronger voices argued in the 1990s in favor of training more generalists, citing among their reasons the growing number of managed care companies that hired generalists to serve as "gatekeepers" to guide enrollees to lower-cost sites for consultation and treatment.

We cannot easily reconcile the views of those who believe in the nation's need for more generalists and their less noisy opponents who concede that some areas have trained more specialists than can be employed. A reasonable resolution is unlikely soon for a variety of reasons. Some believe that the two sides must first clarify whether the United States should cut back on the 16,000 physicians that it has been producing annually, not counting the 30 percent additional international medical graduates who come here for residency training, the vast majority of whom remain to practice. Acknowledging shortages in both selected urban and rural areas, those who believe that the nation has too many physicians agree that it makes limited sense at best to alter the total number of physicians in training and practice. The questions affecting the size of the total physician supply need to be addressed and resolved first.

Even if all concerned could soon reach a consensus regarding the adequacy of the prospective physician supply, including actions to reduce the numbers in training, the resolution of the generalist-specialist distribution would continue to provide a challenge. Generalist preparation is preferred for those who look forward to practicing in a sparsely settled area, where current physician shortages exist. But almost 80 percent of all Americans live in metropolitan areas. Thus, the distribution of the population tends to favor the establishment of multispecialty practices, such as those that currently prevail on the west coast, or smaller group practices that are more prevalent along the east coast, with the rest of the country home to both models.

But important additional issues need to be addressed and re-solved before we can reach a conclusion on this complex and con-fusing health personnel issue. In the early to mid-1990s one heard much about the urgency to train more generalists to meet the growing demands of the rapidly expanding, for-profit managed care plans that were seeking to hire large numbers of generalists to serve as "gatekeepers." And for a brief time generalists' earnings appeared to be rising quite rapidly, which doubtless stimulated increased numbers of medical school seniors to pursue residency training in primary care. But no sooner were these changes in the long-established trends noted and broadcast when the market re-versed. Managed care plans decided to respond to the complaints of many members who saw no point in consulting their gatekeeper before revisiting their specialist who was already treating them for a chronic condition. Further, the earnings differentials between specialists and generalists, which had been narrowing, have again begun to widen.

The pressure to attract and train large numbers of residents in specialty and subspecialty fields is particularly strong in the more important research-oriented AHCs. At these institutions the leadership and the professional staff are heavily committed to treat-ing patients who can profit from high-tech interventions, and the research staff is in turn investigating many complex conditions. Given the focus on sophisticated basic and clinical research, the high proportion of patients that presents serious challenges in both diagnosis and treatment, and the dependence on pursuing sophis-ticated treatments as a major source of revenue, not surprisingly these research-oriented AHCs continue to seek and accept resi-dents who want to pursue residency training in specialty and sub-specialty fields. To a much lesser extent, many research-oriented

AHCs have established or expanded their training of generalists during the past ten years. The AHCs have been able to pursue their objective of providing predominantly specialist training, and this trend reflects the lack of support for more generalist training; at least, the practice opportunities and physician earnings failed to confirm such a need.

As early as the mid-1980s a task force on AHCs, sponsored by the Commonwealth Fund under the chairmanship of Robert Heyssel, former president of The Johns Hopkins Hospital, unanimously recommended that the federal government limit funding for residency training to three years, with five years for persons training for general surgery. The proposal failed to elicit broad support from the leaders of American medicine. The leading AHCs found that the long-term support of the federal government for graduate medical education, some $7 billion annually, has provided an important source of flexible funding for the centers to use to help cross-subsidize activities that do not generate adequate reimbursement. During the debate on the Clinton health care proposal, considerable attention was focused on restructuring the funding and the distribution of these funds, but Congress failed to act on the reform package. The issue has reemerged in connection with the federal executive and legislative commission charged with formulating recommendations about the future financing of Medicare. By 1999 many congressional leaders agreed that sizable savings in graduate medical education funding would be practical, but they faced strong opposition from the leadership of the American Association of Medical Colleges.

One related issue that has been able to engage support of various medical leadership groups concerns the international medical graduates admitted each year for residency training. The American Association of Medical Colleges, the AMA, and congressionally appointed advisory council on health personnel have jointly recommended that the number of these graduates be reduced to not more than 10 percent of U.S. medical school graduates. The advocates for limiting future inflows argue that the country may otherwise have to explore cutbacks in admissions to U.S. medical schools. Indeed, one advisory body has already recommended the closure of about 20 of the 124 allopathic schools currently in operation. This group believes that permitting the large inflow of international graduates to continue in the face of such actions would be irresponsible.

As is the case with most issues of physician personnel policy, the recommendation to reduce the future inflow of international graduates has met with opposition. The few states in which residency training of these graduates is heavily concentrated, such as New York teaching hospitals, depend heavily on this group. Moreover, international graduates often accept positions that U.S. graduates avoid. For example, some international graduates decide to start a permanent practice in underserved areas where they have completed their training. And many within this group serve in various publicly supported and operated institutions, such as state mental hospitals and prisons that usually have difficulty in attracting U.S. medical school graduates. It is difficult to say whether Congress will act on the IMG issue soon or wait to address it as part of the broader issues involved in the future supply of physicians, Most likely Congress will move slowly in restricting the future inflow of IMGs.

In cooperation with a number of leading medical training institutions in New York and in selected other states, HCFA is leading a federal initiative aimed at cutting back the output of residents by about 20 to 25 percent over the course of a five-year demonstration. Many AHCs in New York initially volunteered to participate but later dropped out after discovering that they would have to hire additional personnel while complicating their ability to care for severely ill patients. Among the better-known teaching institutions that had dropped out of the demonstration were Beth Israel Medical Center, Montefiore Medical Center, New York Hospital–Presbyterian Hospital, St. Luke's–Roosevelt Hospital Center.

Having briefly examined several critical interactions between the AHCs and the training of future physicians, we also need to consider some of the new challenges that the AHCs face by virtue of ongoing changes in their patient care environment, specifically the declining average length of stay for inpatient treatment. This number currently ranges from 4 to 6 days, scarcely long enough for residents to become knowledgeable about the conditions that precipitated the patient's admission to the hospital, the steps leading to a definitive diagnosis, and the early effects of the attending physician's therapeutic plan.

Criticisms have been leveled at the AHCs for at least two decades for having focused practically all of their training of medical students and residents on inpatient settings. During a visit to the medical school at the University of Washington in the late 1970s, Eli Ginzberg was surprised that the school had recently entered into an agreement to pay the Puget Sound Health Cooperative for the costs of training its juniors and seniors. He never encountered another arrangement like this one. True, a growing number of specialty boards have recently altered their requirements for certification to include extensive training time in an ambulatory environment. Citing the aging population and increasing numbers of chronically ill living at home, far-sighted medical educators have raised the issue, and some schools have begun to experiment with a team approach to the training of medical students. In particular, trainees require experience in working with a group of diverse practitioners, including generalist and specialist physicians, nurses, physical therapists, dieticians, and rehabilitation specialists as well as others under the general guidance of the physician in charge. Clearly a team approach to the future practice of medicine is easier to outline than it is for the AHCs to implement— and even more difficult for managed care plans and large multispecialty practice groups to partner. But the challenge remains even if effective solutions occur slowly.

As we've discussed, AHCs are under increasing financial pressure because of the declining use of their inpatient facilities; the efforts of managed care companies to reduce the charges that they had previously paid for specific procedures together with lowered payments per diem for inpatient care; the selected declines in Medicare reimbursement rates established by the Balanced Budget Act of 1997; and increased enrollment of Medicaid-eligible individuals in prepaid health care plans aimed at reducing the use of costly inpatient hospital care.

In response to these and other revenue pressures, the leading AHCs have explored a combination of initiatives aimed at moderating their costs and expanding their revenues. Many AHCs eliminated large numbers of middle managers. They also consolidated or closed facilities that were losing money. Many found that they could improve their purchasing relations with suppliers. Some reappraised the liberal policies that they had long pursued in cross-subsidizing high-cost patients, including the amount of charity care that they had historically provided. But early on the AHCs encountered limits in the amount of expenses they could reduce, so they increasingly explored ways to generate more revenue. Most large urban AHCs sought to shore up their admission departments so that many uninsured poor who sought admission could be enrolled in Medicaid. Others explored and established varying networks, affiliations, and even asset-based mergers with smaller and, occasionally, larger hospitals to create a referral source for inpatient admissions or ambulatory patients. Such linkages and alliances also facilitated the removal of unneeded beds and were often reflected in an improved bottom line.

Despite the almost constant focus devoted to stay ahead of vulnerable markets and revenue positions, AHCs still cannot relax. They run expensive institutions and their physicians have long ago acquired a strong preference for the best. But their greatest vulnerability derives from ongoing excess bed capacity, which remains constant and often increases in spite of every effort to bringing their use in greater balance with capacity. As we enter the new century, the capacity-revenue imbalances remain major threats to the leading AHCs. Even though the solutions may not be clear, they likely will emerge slowly and be implemented in the years ahead. The United States is not likely to stand by and let its leading medical institutions go under because of revenue shortfalls. The AHCs have been major contributors to the improved health care to the American people in the past, and they still have much to contribute.

We now shift attention to the urban poor to assess the shift in their relations with AHCs from the implementation of Medicare and Medicaid through the end of the twentieth century. We also examine their potential pattern of interaction for the next 10 years. As noted earlier, after the implementation of Medicare and Medicaid, AHCs, particularly the centers that were sponsored by nonprofit universities and not by state governments, distanced themselves increasingly from their poor neighbors whom they no longer needed to ensure adequate numbers of teaching patients. True, they continued to provide considerable amounts of emergency room and clinic care to this population and admitted reasonable numbers of Medicaid patients who required hospitalization. But many AHCs discouraged the uninsured poor from seeking care at their institution.

With the explosive growth of managed care, selected AHCs, particularly those located in or close to urban ghettos, have adopted a positive view about admitting more Medicaid patients. In fact, this group of patients can be the principal source of inpatient revenues of an inner-city AHC. Responding to the growing importance of Medicaid inpatient revenue, some urban AHCs have explored arrangements with local physicians and HMOs caring for the local poor to enlarge their Medicaid inpatient revenues. For example, after two earlier failed attempts, The Johns Hopkins School of Medicine and hospital, located in a Baltimore ghetto, recently launched its third HMO effort.

Even though the Health of the Public Program, which sought to establish and strengthen ties between selected AHCs and their poor neighbors, had, at best, limited success, at least some AHCs have since become more responsive to issues of population health and the special health problems confronting their low-income neighbors. But given the severe financial pressures that confront most AHCs, the speed and degree of their involvement remains generally modest.

Beyond eleemosynary instincts, other factors point to closer links in the years ahead between urban AHCs and the urban poor. The training environment for medical students and residents re-

mains overwhelmingly inpatient oriented, and this setting is inadequate for generalists and specialists whose careers will start and
mature through the middle of the twenty-first century. As medical
educators gain a greater appreciation of their students' and residents' need for more training in ambulatory settings, AHCs may
enter into new and closer relations with the urban poor who receive
much of their care in exactly those clinical surroundings.

In the next 20 years the AHCs are also likely to broaden their
focus on treating the chronically ill, the vast majority of whom
will be living at home. Given the concentration of low-income
patients living in the inner city, the AHCs may find it essential to
provide opportunities particularly for their residents and clinical
staffs to assess, treat, and monitor increasing numbers of chronic
patients living at home, many of whom will require periodic tests
and treatments in the ambulatory and inpatient facilities of their
neighboring AHC. In fact, the current medical training and practice environments for caring for the chronically ill will likely give
way to a new orientation in which multidiscipline specialists are
led by a physician-in-charge. This trend may ultimately dominate
a large sector of medical practice. Once again the AHCs will confront the challenge of gaining access to these new practice environments, which they may be able to do more readily and effectively
by working collaboratively with their low-income neighbors. In
the final section of this chapter we will briefly explore how possible
changes in the health insurance coverage of the urban (and rural)
poor may speed the creation of new links between them and their
nearby AHCs.

Only prophets can foretell the future, but academics should
speculate about the possible directions of future change in policy
and practice. One such forecast relates to the likely passage, pos-

sibly as early as 2004, of universal health insurance coverage, nearly a century after Theodore Roosevelt first placed it on the nation's political agenda when he ran for reelection as president with the Bull Moose Party in 1912. The question that we must confront is why, after almost a century of this and many other failed efforts, might the country finally be close to passing a national health insurance statute—particularly when most Americans disapprove of enlarging the role of the federal government in major economic issues, let alone one that occupies one-seventh of the U.S. economy and is still growing. The answers are varied:

- The number of uninsured Americans as of 1999 exceeds 43 million, and an estimated 30 additional million lack adequate insurance coverage. Added together these numbers mean that 1 out of every 4 inhabitants in the richest nation in the world is without any or adequate health insurance coverage.
- Asserting that it was intolerable for the United States to ignore mounting barriers preventing essential health care for the poor and uninsured youth in this country, Congress appropriated $24 billion in 1997 to assist the states in funding health insurance coverage for this group.
- Although uninsured or poorly insured Americans usually cannot obtain appropriate access to health care, many within this group have been admitted and treated in state-sponsored AHCs, in nonprofit AHCs, and in other safety-net community hospitals and clinics. But many of the uninsured and poorly insured delay seeking care, and when they do seek it, they generally receive about 60 percent of the level of care provided to adequately insured patients, especially for inpatient treatment.
- The United States is the only advanced economy that has

avoided establishing basic health insurance coverage for the entire population. This situation can be largely explained by the presence of many government-funded hospitals that admit and treat large numbers of the nonpaying or part-paying poor, and the considerable amounts of free or below-cost care that most nonprofit and even for-profit hospitals provide through cross-subsidization by overcharging the well-insured and affluent. But in an era of managed care in which payers closely monitor their contracts and their bills, hospitals and clinics are severely hindered in their ability to continue to subsidize the uninsured. If the number and proportion of the uninsured continues to increase as most experts anticipate, the problem of access will become more acute.

• Fortunately not all signs are downbeat. Most discussions of U.S. health care spending have failed to distinguish between government spending and total spending. Given the popular American belief that large differentials in income and wealth are a mainstay of our dynamic economy, and given widespread opposition to higher tax rates (in fact, the United States has one of the lowest tax burdens of any advanced nation), the discussion about the financing of national health insurance needs to be focused on government outlays, not total spending. Clearly the affluent are entitled to spend as much as they want for any approved or licensed procedure or drug.

• At the beginning of 1999 federal and state appropriations included sufficient funds for health, which, if added to the $100 billion annual tax subsidy for group health insurance coverage, amounted to about $640 billion, or just under 8 percent of the U.S. gross domestic product of $8.2 trillion. Admittedly, we would be unable to make all current federal and state health care funding fungible so that it could be redeployed to finance a system of universal health insurance coverage. Nevertheless, this 8 percent figure is comparable to the amount that most advanced European countries spend on their health care system.

- The major challenge to the future financing of the U.S. health system is to ensure that all Americans have access to essential health care services covered by a system of federal-state health insurance. Americans who want more and presumptively better services can also use their own funds and/or employer benefits to pay for the additional care.

- To ensure that total health care spending does not get out of control, federal and state governments need to cooperate with key profit and nonprofit organizations to establish joint bodies that will explore and inform the electorate about shorter- and longer-term policies aimed at the more efficient use of health resources. These policies would include the rates of spending for biomedical research and development, the future supply of physicians, high-priority objectives in inpatient and ambulatory care facilities (with appropriate responsiveness to geographic differentials), and other related challenges.

We should not fault the American public for its reluctance to expand by orders of magnitude the role of the federal government in health planning and policy in 1994. But something is very much awry if the U.S. electorate continues to avoid passing an all-inclusive health insurance coverage act.

If Congress, preferably in cooperation with the states, passes such a comprehensive insurance statute soon, it would go far to provide the poor with broadened access to mainline health care services and, in turn, improve the revenue position of the AHCs and other teaching and community hospitals that face growing difficulties in continuing to fund their critically important missions. Medicare (with an assist from Medicaid) accomplished exactly that in the years following 1966. Millions of poor elderly who lacked health insurance and adequate income were suddenly welcomed and treated by mainline hospitals and physicians. Providing essential health care insurance coverage for the urban (and rural) poor holds the promise of repeating at least in part the earlier successful intervention and adding significantly to their years of healthy life.

No civilized high-income nation, and surely not the United States, can continue to ignore millions of its citizens and legal immigrants who face ever-greater difficulties in obtaining essential medical care because of lack of private health insurance coverage. With such a large number of the citizenry at risk—a number that is only likely to increase in the years ahead—the nation has no alternative but to move expeditiously to enact essential health care coverage for all. The feasibility of such a needed reform is underscored by the fact that current U.S. government appropriations for health amount to 8 percent of the gross domestic product—virtually the same percentage spent by major European nations on their national health care systems.

Selected Reading

Books

Bodenheimer, T. S., and K. Grumbach. *Understanding Health Policy: A Clinical Approach.* Stamford, Conn.: Appleton and Lange, 1995.

Campion, Frank D. *The AMA and U.S. Health Policy Since 1940.* Chicago: Chicago Review Press, 1984.

Fuchs, Victor. *The Health Economy.* Cambridge, Mass.: Harvard University Press, 1986.

Ginzberg, Eli. *Tomorrow's Hospital: A Look to the Twenty-first Century.* New Haven and London: Yale University Press, 1996.

Ginzberg, Eli, ed. *Critical Issues in U.S. Health Reform.* Boulder, Colo.: Westview Press, 1994.

Ginzberg, Eli, Howard Berliner, and Miriam Ostow. *Improving the Health Care of the Poor: The New York City Experience.* New Brunswick, N.J.: Transaction, 1997.

Ginzberg, Eli, and Anna B. Dutka. *The Financing of Biomedical Research.* Baltimore, Md.: Johns Hopkins University Press, 1989.

Rosenberg, Charles E. *The Care of Strangers: The Rise of America's Hospital System.* New York: Basic Books, 1987.

Starr, Paul. *The Social Transformation of American Medicine.* New York: Basic Books, 1983.

Selected Reading

Stevens, Rosemary. *In Sickness and in Wealth.* New York: Basic Books, 1989.

White, Kerr. *Healing the Schism: Epidemiology, Medicine and the Public's Health.* New York: Springer Verlag, 1991.

Journals

Academic Medicine
Health Affairs
Health Care Financing Review
Hospitals and Health Networks
Inquiry
Journal of the American Medical Association
Modern Healthcare
New England Journal of Medicine

Articles and Reports

Boyd, D. *Medicaid Spending Growth Slows.* The Rockefeller Institute of Government, the Center for the Study of the States, Albany, N.Y., January 1998.

The Commonwealth Fund Task Force on Academic Health Centers Report. *Leveling the Playing Field: Financing the Missions of Academic Health Centers.* New York, May 1997.

Dersan, Lori, and Maggie Fischbusch, eds. *Academic Health Centers and the Community: A Practical Guide for Creating Shared Visions.* Health of the Public Program Office, University of California, San Francisco, 1992.

Evans, J. R. "The 'Health of the Public' Approach to Medical Education." *Academic Medicine* 67(11): 719–723 (1992).

Ginzberg, Eli. "The Future Supply of Physicians." *Academic Medicine* 71: 1147–1153 (1996).

Ginzberg, Eli. "The Changing U.S. Health Care Agenda." *JAMA* 279: 501–504 (1998).

Iglehart, J. K. "Rapid Changes for Academic Medical Centers." *New England Journal of Medicine* 332: 407–411 (1995).

Selected Reading

Innui, T. S. "Partnership for Change." *World Health Forum* 14: 247–249 (1993).

Jones, R. "Academic Medicine: Institutions, Programs and Issues." Association of American Medical Colleges Report, Washington, D.C., February 1997.

Kassirer, J. P. "Academic Medical Centers Under Siege." *New England Journal of Medicine* 331: 1370–1371 (1994).

Kaufman, A. "Resistance to Change Has to Be Overcome in Medical Schools." *World Health Forum* 14: 231–232 (1993).

LaLonde, M. A. *New Perspective on the Health of Canadians.* Ottawa: Information Canada, 1974.

Mullan, F., R. M. Politzer, and C. H. Davis. "Medical Migration and the Physician Workforce: International Medical Graduates and American Medicine." *JAMA* 273:1521–1527 (1995).

Pew Charitable Trusts. *Critical Challenges: Revitalizing the Health Professions for the Twenty-first Century.* UCSF Center for the Health Professions Department, San Francisco, 1995.

Reinhardt, U. "Wanted: A Clearly Articulated Social Ethic for American Health Care." *JAMA* 278(17): 1446–1447 (1997).

Rice, D. P., and C. Hoffman. "Chronic Care in America: A Twenty-first Century Challenge." The Institute for Health and Aging at University of California, San Francisco, and the Robert Wood Johnson Foundation, Princeton, N.J., August 1996.

Rosenbaum, S., K. Maloy, J. Stuber, and J. Darnell. *Initial Findings from a Nationwide Study of Outstationed Medical Enrollment Programs at Federally Qualified Health Centers.* The Center for Health Policy Research at George Washington University, Washington, D.C., February 1998.

Ruzek, J., E. O'Neil, R. Willard, and R. W. Rimel. *Trends in U.S. Funding for Biomedical Research.* The Center for the Health Professions at UCSF and the Pew Scholars Program in the Biomedical Sciences, San Francisco, May 1996.

Schroeder, S. A., J. S. Zones, and J. A. Showstack. "Academic Medicine as a Public Trust." *JAMA* 262(18): 803–812 (1989).

Showstack, J., et al. "Health of the Public: The Academic Response." *JAMA* 267(18): 2497–2502 (May 1992).

Selected Reading

Showstack, J., et al. "Health of the Public: The Private Sector Challenge." *JAMA* 276(13): 1071–1074 (1960).

Stimmel, B. D. "Congress and the International Medical Graduate: The Need for Equity." *Mt. Sinai Journal of Medicine* 63: 359–363 (1996).

Thorpe, K. E. *The Rising Number of Uninsured Workers: An Approaching Crisis in Health Care Financing.* The National Coalition on Health Care, Washington, D.C., October 1997.

Ware, J., M. Bayliss, W. Rogers, M. Kosinski, and A. R. Tarlov. "Differences in Four-Year Health Outcomes for Elderly and Poor, Chronically Ill Patients Treated in HMO and Fee for Service Systems." *JAMA* 276(13): 1039–1047 (1996).

Waterman, R. E., and A. Kaufman, eds. *Health of the Public: A Challenge to Academic Health Centers.* The Pew Charitable Trusts and the Rockefeller Foundation, Health of the Public Program Office, San Francisco, 1993.

Data Sources

American Hospital Association. *Emerging Trends Quarterly Briefs.* Chicago, 1993–1998.

Association of American Medical Colleges. *AAMC Data Book: Statistical Information Related to Medical Education.* Washington, D.C., January 1998.

Council on Graduate Medical Education reports to Congress and the Secretary of Health and Human Services, 1992–1996.

Health Insurance Association of America. *Source Book of Health Insurance Data, 1996.* Washington, D.C., 1997.

Health Systems Research. *The Development of Capitation Rates Under Medicaid Managed Care Programs: A Pilot Study,* Vols. 1 and 2. The Henry J. Kaiser Family Foundation, Washington, D.C., November 1997.

Institute for Health Care Research and Policy. *Medicare Chart Book.* The Henry J. Kaiser Family Foundation, Washington, D.C., June 1997.

Medicare Payment Advisory Commission. *Medicare Payment Policy: Report to the Congress, Volume 1: Recommendations* and *Volume 2: Analytical Papers.* Washington, D.C., March 1998.

National Institute for Health Care Management. *Health Care System Data Source,* 1st ed. Washington, D.C., July 1996.

Selected Reading

Physician Payment Review Commission. *Annual Report to Congress.* Washington, D.C., 1997.

U.S. Bureau of the Census. *Statistical Abstract of the United States: 1997* (117th ed.). Washington, D.C., 1997.

Periodic reports issued by the Congressional Budget Office dealing with health care current expenditures and future projections.

Periodic reports issued by the General Accounting Office related to physician supply and Medicare and Medicaid policies. Washington, D.C., 1994–1997.

Index

Index

Index